DON'T PUT
SEND IT PAC~~KING~~
DID YOU KNOW?

* It's best to slim down . . . Just losing ten pounds relieves each knee of a 30-pound load with every stride you take. So lighten your step . . . exponentially!

* Gosh, it could be gout . . . Arthritis includes over 100 inflammatory diseases. The most common have telltale signs you can spot.

* Boswellia isn't an African country . . . It's an extract from the frankincense tree that relieves pain without undesirable side effects. So do several spices you may have in your home right now!

* Biologics are now available . . . The newest drugs for rheumatoid arthritis can halt this debilitating disease fast. Ask your doctor whether they can help you.

* Meals can heal . . . The right nutritional strategies can stop flare-ups and take off extra pounds at the same time. *Outsmart Arthritis* contains 7 days of menus and dozens of recipes.

* Mind games can outsmart arthritis . . . Techniques such as tai-chi, yoga, meditation, and prayer can improve joint health. Plus, find out how music can tune out pain!

OUTSMART ARTHRITIS

PREVENTION'S™

Outsmart Arthritis

EXPERT-ENDORSED REMEDIES FOR SHORT-TERM RELIEF AND LIFETIME CONTROL

The Editors of *Prevention* Health Books

St. Martin's Paperbacks

PREVENTION'S OUTSMART ARTHRITIS

Copyright © 2003 by Rodale Inc.

Prevention is a registered trademark of Rodale Inc.

The quiz that appears in "Assess Your Joint Health" on pages 7 and 8 is © 2001 by the Arthritis Foundation. Reprinted by permission.

All rights reserved. No part of this book may be used or reproduced in any manner whatsoever without written permission except in the case of brief quotations embodied in critical articles or reviews. For information address Rodale Inc., 33 East Minor Street, Emmaus, PA 18098.

ISBN: 0-312-98811-7

Printed in the United States of America

St. Martin's Paperbacks edition / June 2003

Rodale / St. Martin's Paperbacks are published by St. Martin's Press, 175 Fifth Avenue, New York, NY 10010.

10 9 8 7 6 5 4 3 2 1

Visit us on the web at www.prevention.com

NOTICE

CONTENTS

INTRODUCTION

Not all creatures get arthritis. Bats and sloths, for example, seem immune. Then again, they spend most of their lives hanging upside down. While that may work for them, it's mighty impractical for the rest of us.

Yet short of living in this topsy-turvy fashion, we can't help but expose our joints to the risk of arthritis. This may help explain why it is one of the nation's most common chronic health problems, according to the Arthritis Foundation.

While it is prevalent, arthritis is not inevitable. What's more, you don't have to turn your world upside down to beat it. That's what this book is all about.

For many years, doctors believed that arthritis was a single ailment. Today they know that it takes more than 100 different forms, all with one shared characteristic: They cause inflammation in the joints. In Part I, we'll explore some of the more common forms of the disease. The book focuses primarily on osteoarthritis and rheumatoid arthritis, which account for at least ¹8.5 million cases between them.

Fortunately, more and more doctors and other health care professionals have dedicated themselves to eradicating arthritis. A world without arthritis is hardly a pipe dream. For proof, just turn to Part II, where you'll discover the newest medications that are bringing relief to millions of Americans. If you're curious about other, nondrug treatments that can douse the fire in your joints, you'll find the best—from nutritional and herbal supplements to old-fashioned home remedies—right here.

Of course, while conventional medications and alternative therapies can ease arthritis symptoms, they don't work in a vacuum. They're most effective when incorporated into a healthy lifestyle that combines a sensible diet and moderate physical activity with mind-body healing techniques. You'll find the details in Part III.

Then when you're ready to put together all these pieces, you can turn to Part IV, which features a 7-day plan that goes toe-to-toe with arthritis. You'll learn easy strategies for eating better and exercising more, plus other tips that will help heal arthritic joints and improve your overall health. And don't forget to sample the taste-tempting recipes, all packed with nutrients essential to joint health.

For those moments when you need a little extra motivation to stick with your self-care plan, we suggest reading the personal profiles in Part V. You'll meet some amazing people who have refused to let arthritis become an obstacle in their lives. Their stories are bound to entertain and inspire you.

As these women and men demonstrate, you can lead a vital, independent life even with arthritis. We'll provide all the tools you need. The rest is up to you.

And we know you can do it!

Outsmart
Arthritis

PART I

Arthritis 101

CHAPTER ONE

What Is This Pain?

You feel and look as youthful as ever. But lately, you've noticed some subtle changes. Your knees crackle when you stand up. Your thumbs ache. And your shoulders are all stiff and creaky.

You've scoffed at the notion that you, of all people, could be showing signs of arthritis. Now even you're wondering: Could you?

For many people, the word *arthritis* conjures an image of an elderly person leaning on a cane or struggling to open a jar with stiff fingers. Actually, although the incidence of the condition increases with the years, arthritis can affect anyone at any age—even during childhood. In fact, nearly three of every five people with arthritis are under age 65.

According to the Centers for Disease Control and Prevention (CDC), arthritis is the number one cause of disability in the United States, affecting 43 million Americans. The CDC predicts that number will rise to 60 million by the year 2020.

Fortunately, for those who have the disease, the outlook just keeps getting brighter. Arthritis is not a lifetime sentence to pain and immobility. Much can be done to fight it.

To begin, let's review some arthritis basics—its symptoms, risk factors, diagnosis, treatment options, and prognosis. Armed with this essential information, you'll be able to make informed decisions about your care and keep arthritis from controlling your life.

Q. WHAT IS ARTHRITIS, ANYWAY?

A. The word *arthritis* literally means "joint inflammation." It refers to a group of more than 100 diseases and conditions that cause joint pain, stiffness, and swelling. Left to run its course, arthritis can lead to irreversible joint damage. This is why early diagnosis and treatment matter so much.

Of the many kinds of arthritis, the two most common are osteoarthritis (OA) and rheumatoid arthritis (RA). They produce similar symptoms, but they occur for very different reasons.

Osteoarthritis results from joint overuse and misuse. Over time, the cartilage that cushions and protects a joint breaks down, allowing the bones within the joint to rub against one another. OA most often affects the knees, though it can show up in the hands, hips, and spine. In its earliest stages, it may not produce any symptoms. Only after significant cartilage loss will a person notice severe pain and impaired joint function.

In rheumatoid arthritis, the body's immune system attacks joint tissue, for reasons experts can't explain.

The disease usually begins in the hands, wrists, and feet, before moving on to the shoulders, elbows, and hips. Unlike OA, RA tends to progress symmetrically, affecting the same joint on both sides of the body. Besides pain and stiffness, it may cause fatigue, weakness, low-grade fever, and lumps of inflamed tissue under the skin.

Another key distinction between OA and RA involves the swelling. In RA, it feels soft and squishy. In OA, it's harder and bonier.

Q. WHO GETS ARTHRITIS?

A. While experts know how arthritis works, they've yet to figure out why it occurs in the first place. So they can't say for certain why each form of the disease affects some people but not others.

That said, some factors do appear to increase a person's chances of developing joint problems. They include the following. (To assess your own risk, take the quiz on pages 7 and 8.)

Age. While arthritis can strike at any age, osteoarthritis seems to target those over age 45. That doesn't mean OA is inevitable, however.

Gender. Some 74 percent of all osteoarthritis cases—roughly 15.3 million—occur in women. For rheumatoid arthritis, the proportion is about the same, with 71 percent of all cases—roughly 1.5 million—affecting women.

Family history. While genetics plays a role in all forms of arthritis, it's especially significant in rheumatoid arthritis. A person is much more likely to experience RA if a parent or sibling has it.

Personal history of joint damage. Whether it results from an injury or from chronic strain (as from repetitive hand motions), joint damage can raise a person's risk for osteoarthritis.

Weight problems. Excess pounds are a major risk factor for osteoarthritis, especially in the knees. If you are age 45 or older and of average height, but you weigh more than you should, you could cut your chances of developing OA in your knees by half just by losing 11 or more pounds over the next 10 years.

Inactivity. Evidence suggests that regular exercise helps reduce wear and tear on joints by strengthening surrounding muscles. Strong muscles hold joints in proper alignment.

Q. I COULD BE A CANDIDATE FOR ARTHRITIS. HOW CAN I PROTECT MYSELF?

A. As you might surmise from the above list, you can't do much to change some suspected risk factors for arthritis. But others are very much within your control.

Perhaps your best bet for safeguarding your joints is to slim down if you need to. People tend to associate weight loss with heart health. But it also plays a role in osteoarthritis prevention. Being overweight doesn't cause OA. Instead, it has a domino effect. It encourages a sedentary lifestyle, which limits joint movement, which ultimately stiffens joints.

The good news is, you don't need to shed a lot of pounds to make a difference. Consider that when you're walking, every step forward exerts a force on your knee that's equal to about three times your body

ASSESS YOUR JOINT HEALTH

This quiz, developed by the Arthritis Foundation, could be your first step on the road to healthy, pain-free joints. Simply read each question and mark your response.

Step 1: What's Your Risk?

1. Are you 45 years of age or older?

    Yes   No

2. Have you ever had an injury to your knee(s) severe enough to put you in bed, to force you to use a cane, crutch, or brace, or to require surgery?

    Yes   No

3. Are you more than 10 pounds overweight?

    Yes   No

4. Do you currently participate in (or have you in the past) more than 3 hours a day of heavy physical activities, such as bending, lifting, and carrying items, on a regular basis?

    Yes   No

5. Did you have hip problems that caused you to limp as a child?

    Yes   No

Step 2: What Are Your Symptoms?

6. Has a doctor ever told you that you have arthritis?

    Yes   No

7. During the past 12 months, have you had pain, aching, stiffness, or swelling in or around a joint?

    Yes   No

8. In a typical month, were these symptoms present daily for at least half of the days?

Yes   No

9. Do you have pain in your knee(s) or hip(s) when climbing stairs or walking 2 to 3 blocks (¼ mile) on flat ground?

Yes   No

10. Do you have daily pain or stiffness in your hand joints?

Yes   No

11. Are you presently limited in any way in any activities because of joint symptoms (pain, aching, stiffness, loss of motion)?

Yes   No

12. Because of joint symptoms, rate your ability to do the following (0 = no difficulty; 1 = some difficulty; 2 = much difficulty; 3 = unable to do):

a. Dress yourself, including shoelaces and buttons   0 1 2 3
b. Stand up from a straight, armless chair   0 1 2 3
c. Get in and out of a car   0 1 2 3
d. Open a car door   0 1 2 3

Add up the numbers next to each answer:
a + b + c + d = _____

Step 3: What's Your Score?

If you answered yes to any of questions 1 through 5, you are at risk for arthritis. If you answered yes to two or more of questions 6 through 11, you might have symptoms of arthritis. If you scored a 6 or higher on question 12, you should contact a health-care professional immediately. Otherwise, discuss your symptoms with your health-care professional at your next visit.

weight. So losing just 10 pounds would reduce the load by 30 pounds. Remember, that's with *every step*. Over time, it can really add up.

Another strategy for preventing arthritis, particularly OA, is to stay physically active. As mentioned earlier, regular exercise tones up joint-supporting muscles. It also promotes and preserves flexibility. (You'll learn more about the best activities for healthy joints in Chapter 8.)

Beyond slimming down and staying active, some experts believe you can reduce your risk of all kinds of arthritis by eating a balanced diet that adequately nourishes your joints, muscles, and bones. Indeed, research confirms that omega-3 fatty acids—the beneficial fats found in salmon, mackerel, tuna, and sardines, among other cold-water species of fish— may offer some protection against rheumatoid arthritis. (We'll discuss other dietary strategies in Chapter 7.)

Q. I THINK I ALREADY HAVE ARTHRITIS. WHAT SHOULD I DO?

A. Even if you're showing signs of arthritis, you can take steps to slow and possibly stop the progression of the disease. "Don't listen to the old wives' tales," says Sicy H. Lee, M.D., assistant clinical professor of medicine at New York University School of Medicine and attending physician at the Hospital for Joint Diseases, both in New York City. "Lots of people believe that nothing can be done for arthritis. That just isn't so."

The catch is, you need to get a proper diagnosis

and begin treatment as early as possible. First and foremost, that means seeing a doctor—preferably a family practitioner or an internist. He'll evaluate your symptoms, ask questions about your and your family's medical history (for example, did a parent or grandparent have arthritis?), and conduct a thorough physical examination. If you're overweight or you've been physically inactive, your doctor will take that into account as well.

Currently, no medical test can definitely diagnose osteoarthritis or rheumatoid arthritis. Your doctor may order a blood or urine test to rule out other forms of arthritis. He also may order an X ray of the affected joint—though generally, X rays are more useful in the later stages of arthritis, to detect loss of cartilage or changes in bone.

Q. I CAN TAKE CARE OF MY ARTHRITIS MYSELF. WHY SHOULD I SEE A DOCTOR?

A. Because not all joint pain results from arthritis. Only a doctor can rule out other possible causes of your symptoms.

For example, both bursitis and tendonitis can mimic osteoarthritis. These inflammatory joint conditions tend to surface suddenly, then subside within days or weeks. Likewise, certain viruses can trigger symptoms similar to rheumatoid arthritis, says Melanie J. Harrison, M.D., attending rheumatologist at the Hospital for Special Surgery in New York City. Two common culprits are parvovirus B19, which often passes from school-age children to young mothers, and hepatitis C, which can swell the small joints in the hands. Even the various aches and pains associated with the flu can be mistaken for arthritis.

If your doctor confirms that you have some kind of arthritis, he can not only prescribe medications to relieve your pain but also recommend lifestyle strategies to keep your condition from getting worse. Otherwise, you may face joint replacement surgery or even permanent disability down the road.

Q. SO WHAT SORTS OF ARTHRITIS TREATMENTS ARE AVAILABLE THESE DAYS?

A. For pain relief, medications remain the treatment of choice. They've advanced by leaps and bounds in recent years. You have more options today than ever before. (For profiles of the newest and most common drug therapies, see Chapter 3.)

Of course, while medications help manage your symptoms, they don't address the underlying problems that are causing your symptoms in the first place. That's when lifestyle strategies come into play. Slimming down to a healthy weight, following a regular exercise program, and adopting a nutritionally balanced diet not only help prevent arthritis but also preserve and improve the mobility of arthritic joints.

Q. BUT WON'T ALL THAT EXERCISE DO MORE HARM THAN GOOD?

A. On the contrary! If you want to ease your pain, enhance your flexibility, reduce your reliance on medications, and possibly avoid joint replacement surgery, then you *must* get moving, says Justus J. Fiechtner,

M.D., M.P.H., head of rheumatology at Michigan State University in East Lansing. "Medications may take away the pain," he explains, "but if you don't engage in some form of exercise, you'll never increase your strength and, therefore, your function." Some studies have shown that aerobic activities such as walking actually fight inflammation in certain joints.

For his patients with osteoarthritis, Dr. Fiechtner writes a fitness "prescription" that includes aerobic activity, strengthening exercises, and stretching. The same sort of program may help in cases of rheumatoid arthritis, though with this form of arthritis, you must be sure to rest your joints during periods of active inflammation.

Q. HOW WILL STRETCHING HELP MY JOINTS?

A. When you have pain in one of your joints, you may be reluctant to move it. But the less active it is, the stiffer it becomes. Over time, even the most routine tasks—like retrieving a can from the top shelf of the pantry or turning your head to back up your car—could prove unbearable.

With regular stretching, you improve your flexibility and expand your range of motion. So you increase your chances of staying active and independent, despite your arthritis.

Q. WHAT ABOUT STRENGTH TRAINING? HOW WILL IT HELP?

A. As we discussed previously, exercise builds muscle, and muscle supports joints. But only strength training will do the job. Aerobic activity, while great for mobilizing your joints (and for promoting overall fitness), doesn't target muscle as strength training can.

Actually, if you haven't been exercising regularly, you may need to do some strength training before you try other kinds of physical activity, says William J. Arnold, M.D., rheumatologist and director of the complementary medicine program at the Illinois Bone and Joint Institute in Des Plaines. It will prime your joints for movement and safeguard them against injury.

If you're new to strength training, your best bet is to work with a physical therapist or personal trainer to develop a joint-friendly workout and learn proper form. You can use free weights or machines, or you can go with a less-conventional option, like elastic bands. Choose whatever you're most comfortable with.

Q. WE'VE TALKED ABOUT MEDICATIONS AND LIFESTYLE STRATEGIES. DO ANY ALTERNATIVE THERAPIES SHOW PROMISE FOR EASING ARTHRITIS SYMPTOMS?

A. Absolutely! An ever-growing body of research suggests that a number of alternative therapies offer safe, effective relief from arthritis pain. For example, certain nutritional supplements have proven useful in repairing protective cartilage and preventing oxidative damage to joints (see Chapter 4). And certain herbs hold their own against conventional pharmaceuticals in fighting inflammation (see Chapter 5).

With these and other alternative therapies, you do need to exercise some caution. Some make claims that just don't hold up with further study. Some may adversely interact with any conventional medications that are part of your self-care plan. For these reasons, you ought to discuss any alternative therapies with your doctor or another qualified health care professional before you decide to try them.

Q. WILL WE EVER SEE A CURE FOR ARTHRITIS?

A. According to John Klippel, M.D., medical director of the Atlanta-based Arthritis Foundation, scientists must determine what causes arthritis and how the body reacts to the resulting damage before they figure out how to stop the disease. "Finding a cure by serendipity seems highly unlikely," Dr. Klippel notes.

Currently, some of the most promising research centers on the role of genetics in determining a person's risk of joint problems. "Which genes are involved, and what they make or don't make, is key," Dr. Klippel says. "For example, while I may have genes that protect against arthritis, someone else may have genes that increase susceptibility to the disease."

That's not to suggest lifestyle factors don't matter. They do—perhaps even more so for a person with a genetic predisposition to arthritis. The point is, Dr. Klippel says, "If we're going to start using this word *cure*, we're going to need to make a real investment in research."

Q. SO WHAT IS THE OUTLOOK FOR PEOPLE WITH ARTHRITIS?

A. "I've been working in arthritis research for more than 16 years," says Leigh F. Callahan, Ph.D., asso-

GO AHEAD—GET CRACKIN'

So does cracking your knuckles really lead to arthritis?

As far as the experts can tell, no. That's according to Teresa J. Brady, Ph.D., medical adviser for the Atlanta-based Arthritis Foundation.

Dr. Brady frequently was asked the same question when she gave presentations on arthritis. "I'd answer by saying, 'Your grandmother probably told you not to do it, and probably because it annoyed her,'" Dr. Brady says.

As for the source of the cracking sound, experts have a couple of explanations. One is that pressing on the knuckles bursts tiny air bubbles in the synovial fluid of the finger joints— kind of like cracking bubbles in gum. Another is that tendons snap over a little outcropping of bone.

While overuse and misuse of a joint can lead to arthritis, cracking knuckles tends to be a "moment in time" pressure on the joint, not a continuous strain. "If someone does it a couple of times a day, every day, I wouldn't be concerned," Dr. Brady says. "It probably won't increase the person's risk of arthritis. But it may annoy those nearby."

ciate director of the Thurston Arthritis Research Center at the University of North Carolina at Chapel Hill. "Things are changing. We have a good feeling about where we are in terms of arthritis treatment."

"We don't see as many wheelchairs in our clinics as in the past," Dr. Harrison confirms. "Fewer people come in with contracted hands and deformed fingers." Part of the reason, she says, is that doctors are prescribing potent new medications with fewer side effects. These medications, known as DMARDs (for disease-modifying antirheumatic drugs), not only reduce inflammation but also seem to slow the advance of arthritis. In addition, they address more serious complications, like muscle wasting and joint contraction from disuse, Dr. Harrison says.

Of course, alternative therapies continue to gain ground as legitimate arthritis treatments. Not so long ago, few Americans would have considered seeing anyone other than a conventionally trained physician for their arthritis pain. Today more and more people are exploring options outside mainstream medicine, encouraged by positive research findings and their own good results.

Beyond medications and alternative therapies, an array of adaptive tools exists to simplify various tasks for swollen, painful joints. These tools range from kitchen utensils with large, padded handles for easier gripping to gadgets for buttoning and unbuttoning shirts.

In short, a diagnosis of arthritis doesn't mean an end to active living. Instead, it's the beginning of an action plan for a vital, independent life.

CHAPTER TWO

The Many Faces of Arthritis

While osteoarthritis and rheumatoid arthritis account for the vast majority of arthritis cases, they're just two of more than 100 variations on the condition. We couldn't possibly cover all of them in so little space. But we can showcase a handful that merit extra attention, for one reason or another.

Think of arthritis as the trunk of a rather large family tree. Some forms of the condition branch out in a very predictable manner, like dependable Aunt Martha. Others grow in wildly different directions, like eccentric Cousin Earl. They're the ones that might easily be misunderstood or overlooked as members of the arthritis family. You'll get to know them here.

FIBROMYALGIA: WHEN YOU HURT ALL OVER

People who develop fibromyalgia often confuse it with the flu, at least in the beginning. Both conditions produce a characteristic all-over achiness. Only in fibromyalgia, it doesn't go away after a week or two. It can linger for months, years, or even decades.

Experts don't know for sure what causes fibromyalgia. One theory is that it stems from injuries affecting the central nervous system—which may explain why it shows up in a large percentage of whiplash victims. Another theory is that fibromyalgia results from changes in muscle metabolism, which could contribute to diminished blood flow and fatigue.

Some evidence suggests that fibromyalgia may be triggered by bacterial or viral infections. Research has found that the condition occurs in 10 to 25 percent of people with Lyme disease, a bacterial infection that's transmitted by ticks. (We'll talk more about Lyme disease later in the chapter.)

Telltale Signs

According to estimates, between 3 million and 6 million Americans have fibromyalgia. It's most common in women in their childbearing years, but it can affect anyone of any age.

Perhaps the best-known symptom of fibromyalgia is the so-called tender points. These extremely sensitive areas tend to crop up in the neck, shoulders, spine, and hips, says Lenore Buckley, M.D., professor of internal medicine and pediatrics at the Virginia Commonwealth University Medical College of Virginia in Richmond.

Another common symptom is poor sleep. Not that people with fibromyalgia don't get enough: Most say they snooze for 10 or more hours a night. The problem is, they don't achieve the deeper stages of sleep that they need to feel refreshed. This can leave them feeling groggy and "out of it" when they wake up in the morning. It also can interfere with their ability to concentrate during the day.

Besides tender points and poor sleep, people with fibromyalgia often report muscle stiffness, headaches, depression, and an overwhelming sense of fatigue. They may be too tired to perform even the simplest daily activities.

Because any of these symptoms could occur with some other condition, diagnosing fibromyalgia can be a challenge. You're a likely candidate if you experience tender points and widespread pain for more than 3 months, and tests confirm that your symptoms are not caused by rheumatoid arthritis, lupus, or Lyme disease.

Taking Control

While experts have yet to find a cure for fibromyalgia, that's no reason to let the condition take over your life. For most people, it tends to occur in spurts, with occasional flare-ups followed by periods of remission. Sometimes it goes away as spontaneously as it came.

At the very least, you can take steps to control the frequency and severity of your flare-ups. Here's what to do.

For Immediate Relief
Get as much exercise as you can. Walking, cycling, and other forms of physical activity help reduce muscle pain and tenderness. They also stimulate the production of endorphins, chemical messengers in the

brain that promote feelings of relaxation and well-being.

Even with the benefits of exercise as motivation, launching a fitness routine can be difficult, especially when you have fibromyalgia. Your muscles already feel sore and achy. But if you can push through the initial discomfort, you'll be glad you did. As your muscles grow stronger, your symptoms will diminish. Plus, you'll notice increases in energy and endurance.

If you haven't been physically active, you'll want to start with some simple stretching exercises before advancing to a full-fledged workout. For an intermediate activity, try walking, Dr. Buckley says. Start with 5 minutes and gradually increase your time and intensity until you're walking briskly for 40 minutes three days a week.

Sign up for aqua-aerobics. "Warm-water exercises are very beneficial for fibromyalgia, because they relax muscles and decrease pain," Dr. Buckley says. "The water supports your body, so you're not working against gravity."

While you can head for the nearest pool and work out on your own, you're better off enrolling in a class designed especially for people with fibromyalgia. "You want to be sure that you're doing the moves correctly, so you don't hurt yourself," Dr. Buckley explains. Your doctor may be able to provide a referral to a physical therapy clinic that offers aqua-aerobics classes. Or check with local health clubs and YM/YWCAs. Many sponsor classes in cooperation with the Arthritis Foundation.

Treat your body to yoga. Even though regular exercise can help ease fibromyalgia symptoms, some people with the condition may feel too tired or sore for physical activity. If you're in this group, yoga may be your best choice. It's gentle and low-impact, yet it primes your muscles with a good workout.

One caveat: If you're new to yoga, you need to get some basic instruction in proper form and technique—ideally, in a beginner-level class. Many health clubs and YM/YWCAs offer them.

Steer clear of caffeine. Coffee, tea, and other caffeine-containing beverages are America's favorite pick-me-ups. But people tend to forget just how stimulating caffeine can be. Consumed too close to bedtime, it can disrupt the deep, restorative sleep that's already in short supply in cases of fibromyalgia.

Try to limit yourself to one or two servings of caffeine-containing beverages a day. Avoid them altogether in the afternoon and evening.

Medical Options
Consider antidepressants for pain relief and more. Even if you don't have depression, antidepressant medications like amitriptyline (Elavil or Endep) and fluoxetine (Prozac) may help manage your fibromyalgia. Aside from reducing muscle pain, they also improve sleep and increase energy, which in turn may encourage a more active lifestyle.

Ask your doctor about combining drugs. In a study at Newton-Wellesley Hospital in Newton, Massachusetts, people with fibromyalgia were given Elavil, Prozac, or a combination of the two drugs. Those who took the combination experienced twice as much improvement in their symptoms as those who took just one of the drugs.

Researchers suspect that the combination of Elavil and Prozac may change the perception of pain in people with fibromyalgia. The medications affect blood flow to pain-receptive regions of the brain. They also enhance the production of serotonin and other feel-good chemicals.

To Stay on Top of Your Symptoms
Adopt a positive mindset. Being optimistic and upbeat is a tall order when you're hurting. But it's worth the effort. Studies have shown that people who dwell on their pain experience a lot more stress, which in turn increases their pain.

In one large study, researchers at the University of Missouri in Columbia compared drug and nondrug treatments for fibromyalgia. They found that people who engaged in regular exercise or practiced cognitive-behavioral therapy—which involves replacing negative thoughts with positive ones—reported less pain and fatigue. They also had an easier time performing daily tasks, compared with the people who only took drugs.

You can learn cognitive-behavioral therapy by working with a qualified therapist. But you may get good results simply by setting aside time each day to rest, unwind, and regroup. You can use this time to practice deep breathing or meditation, listen to music, engage in prayer—whatever helps bring about deep, restorative relaxation.

For More Information

- Arthritis Foundation: www.arthritis.org
- Fibromyalgia Network: www.fmnetnews.com

- National Institute of Arthritis and Musculo-skeletal and Skin Diseases: www.niams.nih.gov

GOUT: TOE THE LINE ON PAIN

Of all the forms of arthritis, gout may be the most painful. It results from the buildup of uric acid in the blood. Uric acid is a waste product formed by the breakdown of proteins, particularly those known as purines. This is why people who eat lots of purine-rich foods, like shellfish and organ meats, are at high risk for gout.

Then again, some people develop gout simply because they have a genetic tendency to produce abnormally high amounts of uric acid, or because their bodies can't eliminate it efficiently. "Often gout is inherited," notes Elizabeth Tindall, M.D., associate clinical professor of medicine at Oregon Health Sciences University in Portland. So if someone in your family has it, you're more likely to get it, too.

Other risk factors for gout include having a personal history of kidney disease or high blood pressure, drinking large amounts of alcohol, and eating too many rich foods. In fact, because of its association with decadent behaviors, gout once was known as the rich man's disease. (It is much more common among men than women.)

Telltale Signs

When uric acid reaches high concentrations, it forms sharp crystals that literally stab into joints, often in the big toe. This leads to intense inflammation. "During an acute attack, the joint will be red, hot, and painful," Dr. Tindall says. "Some of my patients have said that they couldn't walk. They couldn't stand to have a bed sheet touching the affected foot."

The onset of gout can be sudden and unexpected. Uric acid can quietly stockpile for years and years, only to painfully announce its presence in the middle of the night. Typically, the pain lasts a day or two. But it can feel like forever.

Taking Control

Once you've lived through one attack of gout, you'll never want to experience another. The following strategies can put a quick end to your pain and keep it from coming back.

For Immediate Relief

Pamper your foot. As mentioned above, while gout can affect just about any joint, it usually targets the big toe. Dr. Tindall recommends taking all the weight off the affected foot by removing your shoe and sock and lying on your bed. But skip the sheets and blankets; even they can cause pain if they touch your toe.

Apply ice—or heat. People respond to cold and heat treatments differently, Dr. Tindall says. You need to experiment to find which one works best for you.

Cold can help because it reduces swelling. Try wrapping some ice cubes in a washcloth and holding them against your toe for 10 or 15 minutes.

If you're not comfortable with the cold sensation, you can switch to heat. Wrap a hot water bottle in a towel and apply it to your toe. Or use a heating pad.

Medical Options
Go over-the-counter first. At the onset of a gout attack, take ibuprofen or another over-the-counter pain reliever, Dr. Tindall advises. These drugs help curtail the body's production of prostaglandins, chemicals that cause pain and inflammation. But stay away from aspirin. It can block the excretion of uric acid by the kidneys, making a gout attack even worse.

Choose colchicine for prescription-strength relief. Colchicine can stop the pain of gout within an hour or two. But it works best if it's taken within 12 hours of the onset of an attack. If you wait much longer than that, it won't be as effective.

Save corticosteroids as a last resort. Given orally or by injection, corticosteroids are considered the "gold standard" for stopping inflammation. But because they can produce serious side effects, these powerful drugs should be used only when other treatments don't work.

To Prevent Another Attack
Stay away from alcohol. "Alcohol is the number-one dietary contributor to gout, because it interferes with the kidneys' ability to excrete uric acid," Dr. Tindall says. Some people can get away with drinking small amounts of alcohol, but most are better off giving it up altogether.

Weed purines from your diet. Besides shellfish and organ meats, food sources of purines include anchovies and red meats. Of course, women may need to eat some red meat in order to fulfill their bodies' iron requirements. "I recommend keeping the serving to about the size of a deck of playing cards," Dr.

Tindall says. "Eating that much red meat twice a week is fine."

Drink lots of water. Water increases the amount of uric acid excreted by the kidneys, Dr. Tindall explains. Drinking up is especially important when you've been exercising or working hard, as dehydration can trigger a gout attack. Aim for six to eight 8-ounce glasses a day—more when you're active.

Maintain a healthy weight. If you weigh more than you should, losing any extra pounds can reduce the amount of uric acid produced by your body. That cuts your chances of a future gout attack.

So what's the secret to slimming down successfully? Actually, it isn't much of a secret: Eat healthfully and exercise regularly.

"If you limit red meat, you'll automatically consume less fat and fewer calories, along with cutting down on purines," Dr. Tindall notes. You can build your diet around nutrient-packed plant foods—fruits, vegetables, legumes, and whole grains.

As for exercise, Dr. Tindall advises her patients to engage in some form of aerobic activity—such as jogging, cycling, swimming, or aerobic dance—most days of the week. If you've been relatively sedentary, remember to ease into your fitness routine, gradually increasing the intensity and duration of your workouts.

For More Information

- Arthritis Foundation: www.arthritis.org
- National Institute of Arthritis and Musculo-skeletal and Skin Diseases: www.niams.nih.gov

LUPUS: IMMUNITY GONE AWRY

Lupus is what's known as an autoimmune disorder. This means the immune system turns on the body, attacking perfectly healthy tissues for no apparent reason. In lupus, it seems to target the connective tissue, causing inflammation. Determining just how many Americans have lupus is something of a challenge, since the symptoms of the condition can vary so widely—even for the same person over time. Studies have shown that lupus affects 8 to 10 times as many women as men. Usually it strikes during the child-bearing years, though some women are older when they get it.

Researchers have yet to figure out why women are at such higher risk. They're looking into a possible hormone connection, particularly involving estrogen. Other suspected causes of lupus include bacterial and viral infections and exposure to certain environmental toxins—though which toxins they are and exactly what role they play remain to be seen.

Telltale Signs

Lupus is known as the disease with a thousand faces because it causes such an incredible range of symptoms—from fatigue, achiness, and swollen joints to persistent fever, anemia, rashes, and sensitivity to sunlight. In severe cases, it can damage the heart, lungs, kidneys, and other vital organs.

Currently, no single test can diagnose lupus. If you're showing symptoms of the condition, your doctor may run what's known as an immunofluorescent antinuclear antibody (ANA) test. A positive result on this blood test doesn't mean you have lupus; other diseases and some medications can cause false-positives. In fact, only a relative handful of patients with antinuclear antibodies actually have lupus. So why even run the test? Because almost everyone who has lupus gets positive results on it.

Your doctor also may order a blood test to check your erythrocyte sedimentation rate. This is the speed at which your red blood cells settle to the bottom of the test tube. A faster-than-normal speed could indicate a systemic disease like lupus.

Your doctor may assess your blood count, too. People with lupus tend to register low numbers for white blood cells. Low levels of blood platelets and hemoglobin also may be indicators of lupus.

Taking Control

Because lupus causes so many symptoms and is so unpredictable—sudden flare-ups followed by long periods of remission—it doesn't come with a one-size-fits-all treatment plan. You and your doctor need to determine which strategies will work best for your particular situation. Use the following as your starting point.

For Immediate Relief
Get plenty of rest. Physical exhaustion is among the most common symptoms of lupus. It also can trigger a flare-up. For these reasons, getting a good night's sleep every night is one of the most important mea-

sures for effectively managing your condition. It's also beneficial to your immune system, as your body may use your sleep time to repair cellular damage, according to Michael Lockshin, M.D., director of the Barbara Volcker Rheumatology Center at the Hospital for Special Surgery in New York City.

Medical Options

Treat symptoms with an over-the-counter anti-inflammatory. Many people with lupus experience joint pain and swelling, which can significantly reduce their ability to get around. Aspirin and ibuprofen help relieve inflammation as well as pain, Dr. Lockshin says.

Use meds to rein in your immune system. When lupus is "active," the immune system can literally destroy tissue throughout the body. Sooner or later, your doctor will probably prescribe medications to suppress immunity and alleviate inflammation and pain. Among the most common pharmaceutical treatments for lupus are corticosteroids, azathioprine (Imuran), and cyclophosphamide (Cytoxan). All of these can be very effective, but they also are rife with side effects.

If your doctor prescribes corticosteroids, the dosage will likely be tapered over time. This process gradually weans your body from the medication without causing any adverse effects. The other drugs don't require tapering.

To Minimize Future Flare-ups

Eat well. While no specific dietary guidelines exist for lupus, following a well-balanced diet is essential for a healthy immune system. Generally, doctors ad-

vise people with lupus to restrict their consumption
of red meat and other fatty foods, instead building
their meals around a variety of whole grains, legumes,
fruits, and vegetables. This is a sound strategy for
everyone, regardless of whether they have lupus, Dr.
Lockshin notes.

Exercise as much as you're able. Many people
with lupus are so tired and achy that the very thought
of working out could bring on the urge to take a nap.
But staying active is important, especially in cases of
lupus. It promotes a sense of physical and emotional
well-being.

Before you launch an exercise program, ask your
doctor or a physical therapist to recommend a workout that's appropriate for your situation. Some of the
best activities are walking, cycling, and swimming.
You probably should avoid pounding exercises such
as running, which put extra stress on already tender
joints.

Be smart about sun exposure. About one-third
of people with lupus are extremely sensitive to the
sun, Dr. Lockshin says. Even a small amount of sun
exposure could trigger a flare-up.

Dr. Lockshin recommends staying out of the sun
between 10 A.M. and 3 P.M., when the rays are their
strongest. Try to plan outdoor activities for first thing
in the morning or later in the evening. And when you
are outside, wear a sunscreen with an SPF of at least
15, he advises. Be sure to reapply often—especially
if you're swimming or perspiring, both of which will
wash the sunscreen off your skin.

Find ways to short-circuit stress. People with
lupus seem more vulnerable to flare-ups when they're

going through difficult times. "Everyone experiences stress, but people with lupus really should try to avoid it," Dr. Lockshin says.

Some of his patients have asked about practicing stress-reduction techniques such as deep breathing, meditation, yoga, and biofeedback. Since these can be helpful, he usually urges anyone who wants to try them to go ahead.

If you need help coping with a particularly stressful situation, you may want to consider professional counseling. Support groups for people with lupus also exist. To find one in your area, check with your doctor or local hospital.

Treat colds and flu immediately. Even though lupus involves an overzealous immune system, people with this condition are *more* susceptible to infections, including colds and flu. And when they get sick, they may need more time to recover.

Of course, avoiding cold and flu viruses is next to impossible. And because certain treatments for lupus may inhibit the immune system, fighting an infection can be all the more difficult. Your best bet is to see your doctor as soon as you notice any symptoms. Even a seemingly minor infection can be much more serious when you're dealing with lupus.

For More Information

• Lupus Foundation of America: www.lupus.org

LYME DISEASE: OUTWIT THOSE TICKS

Ever since the first widely publicized outbreak of Lyme disease—an acute inflammatory disease—in

1975, many Americans have shied away from hiking in woods, fields, and other areas inhabited by deer ticks. They're the bugs responsible for transmitting the sometimes painful bacterial infection.

You have every reason to take precautions against Lyme disease, especially if you live in a high-risk region, such as the Northeast, the Upper Midwest, or the Pacific Coast states. By the same token, you shouldn't limit your outdoor activities because of it. "This country has a lot of unwarranted anxiety about Lyme disease," observes Robert T. Schoen, M.D., a leading Lyme disease researcher and clinical professor of medicine at Yale University School of Medicine in New Haven, Connecticut.

The number of ticks that actually carry the Lyme bacterium varies considerably by region. Less than 5 percent of adult ticks south of Maryland have it, compared with up to 50 percent in some areas of the Northeast.

Telltale Signs

In general, people don't realize they've been exposed to the Lyme bacterium until they develop symptoms of infection. Perhaps the best-known symptom is the telltale skin rash that looks like a bull's-eye. Others include joint pain, fever, and fatigue.

Taking Control

If you are bitten by a deer tick, it doesn't mean that you're going to develop Lyme disease. The actual transmission of the Lyme bacterium from a tick to a human takes more than 24 hours. The following steps can help reduce your chances of infection.

For Immediate Relief
Remove ticks as quickly as possible. Ticks that haven't started feeding can be flicked off the skin with a washcloth or towel. Once they're embedded in the skin, however, they really hang on. That's when your risk for developing Lyme disease begins to rise.

To remove a tick, grip it close to the skin with a pair of tweezers and pull on it with gentle, steady pressure. It should pop right out. Try not to squeeze the body, which could inject Lyme bacterium into your skin. Afterward, wash your hands, the bite, and the tweezers with soap and water to disinfect them.

Medical Options
Kill the bacteria with antibiotics. For all the worry about Lyme disease, most cases are very treatable. If you're diagnosed with the disease, your doctor probably will prescribe a course of antibiotics, typically amoxicillin or doxycycline. That should be enough to knock out the infection for good.

Prevent infection with a vaccine. Researchers have developed a vaccine that reduces the risk of Lyme infection in people between ages 15 and 70 by about 78 percent. Those who live in tick-infested areas and engage in activities that may raise their risk should consider the vaccine, Dr. Schoen says. It isn't foolproof, but it will provide significant protection.

The vaccine is administered as a series of three shots over a 12-month period. "Studies have shown that 's safe and effective," Dr. Schoen adds. Talk with your doctor to assess your individual risk and determine whether you might benefit from the vaccine.

To Reduce Your Risk of Tick Bites

Wear appropriate outdoor attire. If you live in an area that's known to harbor deer ticks, slip on a long-sleeved shirt and pants before you head outside. Choose light-colored garments, so you can easily spot any ticks that happen to climb on board. Tuck your pants into your socks or boots to keep the bugs from finding your legs.

Use insect repellent. For extra protection, be sure to spray insect repellent on your clothing and any exposed skin before stepping out the door. Look for a product containing 20 to 30 percent diethyltoluamide, or DEET—one of the most effective ingredients on the market. Be aware that repellents of this strength are for adults only. For children over age 2, choose a product with no more than 10 percent DEET—and check with your pediatrician before using it. Never apply repellents containing DEET to children age 2 and under.

Stay out of high-risk areas. You really don't need to stay inside during tick season, which usually runs from May through July. But do try to steer clear of favorite tick habitats—especially moist, shady areas with a groundcover of leaves or low-lying vegetation.

Keep up with yard maintenance. Even if your home is in the suburbs, deer ticks could be lurking close by. You can keep them from getting too cozy by cutting your grass short and clearing leaves and brush from around your yard.

If you live in a heavily wooded area, you may want to thin the trees to allow in more sunlight. This cuts down on ticks by reducing the available habitat for the deer and mice that carry the pests.

For More Information

- Centers for Disease Control and Prevention: www.cdc.gov

PART II

Choosing Treatments

CHAPTER THREE

The Arthritis Super Drugs

Arthritis is nothing new. Heck, even dinosaurs showed signs of joint problems. Unfortunately for them, they couldn't take advantage of all the medications that we have today. And more are on the way, as researchers continue their work on groundbreaking new treatments that might put arthritis . . . well, on the "extinct" list.

In this chapter, we'll take a closer look at some of the most popular drug therapies for osteoarthritis and rheumatoid arthritis. While these medicines won't cure joint problems, they can relieve pain and help prevent long-term disability. One of them may have a place in your self-care plan.

RELIEF FOR OSTEOARTHRITIS

For years, Sarah Huffman had to choose between joint pain and stomach pain. Diagnosed with osteoarthritis while in her fifties, Huffman tried a variety of phar-

maceutical treatments before finding one that eased
the ache in her legs and feet. But this particular medication—a traditional nonsteroidal anti-inflammatory
drug (NSAID)—also upset her stomach.

Traditional NSAIDs such as aspirin, ibuprofen, ke-
toprofen, and naproxen sodium—the most commonly
used osteoarthritis medicines in the United States—
do a good job of easing the pain, inflammation, and
stiffness that accompany the disease. But they can
cause assorted side effects, including gastrointestinal
problems that range from stomach pain to ulcers and
bleeding. When the medications are taken only occasionally, the risk of side effects is small. But it
grows with the duration of the treatment and the size
of the dose. Those who are older or who have other
health problems are at particular risk. "Because of
that, my doctor told me to use my medication only
when the pain was bad," says Huffman, now a retiree
living in Fairfield, Virginia.

Then her doctor switched her to one of a new group
of NSAIDs called COX-2 inhibitors. At last, Huffman
found no-strings-attached relief. "It's been great for
me," she says. "I have much less pain and no stomach
problems."

Know Your Options

The odds that you'll find maximum relief from osteoarthritis symptoms—with minimal side effects—are
better than ever these days, thanks to a number of
drug therapies that have hit the market in recent years.
"If the medication you're taking isn't working, or if
it's causing side effects, there's a good chance that

another drug will be a better match," says John Klippel, M.D., medical director of the Atlanta-based Arthritis Foundation. Review the following options, and discuss them with your doctor.

Celecoxib (Celebrex), Rofecoxib (Vioxx), Valdecoxib (Bextra)

The benefits: In studies, these drugs—collectively known as COX-2 inhibitors, or COX-2s—have proven as effective as traditional NSAIDs in relieving inflammation and pain. But they're less likely to cause gastrointestinal side effects. "They're an important advance because they're safer, particularly for people who have experienced gastrointestinal complications," Dr. Klippel says.

The COX-2s also are less likely than traditional NSAIDs to boost your susceptibility to bruising and bleeding. That's because they don't thin your blood—that is, reduce clotting—as the older medications do, explains Roland Moskowitz, M.D., professor of medicine at Case Western Reserve University Medical School in Cleveland. Some preliminary studies suggest that the COX-2s may offer some protection against colon cancer.

Traditional NSAIDs work by blocking two enzymes—one called COX-1 and the other, COX-2. The COX-2 enzyme plays a role in osteoarthritis, while COX-1 helps protect the stomach and kidneys and regulates blood flow. That's why traditional NSAIDs can cause gastrointestinal problems and raise the risk of bleeding. And it's why the newer COX-2 inhibitors—which target COX-2 but pretty much ignore COX-1—are less likely to produce adverse effects.

The drawbacks: Because the COX-2s don't thin the blood, they don't prevent blood clots as traditional NSAIDs can. So they won't help reduce the risk of heart attack or stroke. And while they're less likely than traditional NSAIDs to cause gastrointestinal trouble, they still produce other similar side effects: dizziness, drowsiness, fluid retention, impaired kidney function, rashes, ringing in the ears, and—in high doses—liver problems.

Be aware, too, that some insurers will cover the cost of the COX-2s only if you've experienced problems with traditional NSAIDs.

They may be right for you if . . . you're at increased risk for gastrointestinal upset, ulcers, and bleeding. Some experts, including Dr. Moskowitz, go one step farther. They recommend COX-2s for *everyone*, because the drugs are safer than traditional NSAIDs.

They may not be right for you if . . . you have kidney problems. Research has yet to determine whether the COX-2s are easier on the kidneys than traditional NSAIDs, says Hani El-Gabalawy, M.D., director of the Arthritis Centre at the University of Manitoba in Winnipeg. The same caution applies if you have very high blood pressure, since the kidneys help to regulate blood pressure.

You also need to be careful with the COX-2s if you have heart disease. Some research suggests that traditional NSAIDs can raise the risk of congestive heart failure in older people with heart disease. Whether COX-2s produce the same effect isn't clear.

If you're allergic to NSAIDs, you may not be able to take COX-2s, either. Ask your doctor.

Variations: Chemically, celecoxib is similar in structure to sulfonamide, or sulfa drugs. If you're allergic to these drugs, you may not be able to tolerate celecoxib, either. Rofecoxib has a different structure, so it's a good alternative.

For maximum effectiveness: Do not mix COX-2s with other prescription or over-the-counter NSAIDs.

Meloxicam (Mobic)

The benefits: Meloxicam is as effective against inflammation and pain as traditional NSAIDs. But it's easier on the gastrointestinal tract, Dr. Klippel says.

The drawbacks: Meloxicam doesn't seem to be as easy on the gastrointestinal tract as rofecoxib or celecoxib, particularly in larger doses. Though it is sometimes classified as a COX-2 inhibitor, meloxicam acts more like a traditional NSAID. With the exception of gastrointestinal problems, its side effects are similar to those of traditional NSAIDs.

It may be right for you if . . . you're not getting good results from celecoxib or rofecoxib, and you're at risk for gastrointestinal trouble. In that case, a low dose of meloxicam may be an effective alternative, Dr. Moskowitz says.

It may not be right for you if . . . you're at high risk for gastrointestinal side effects and you need a large dose of meloxicam to get osteoarthritis relief. Your best bet may be to try another medication.

Diclofenac Sodium/Misoprostol (Arthrotec)

The benefits: Arthrotec pairs the traditional NSAID diclofenac sodium with misoprostol, which helps protect the gastrointestinal tract. For this reason, Arthrotec is less likely than traditional NSAIDs to cause gastrointestinal problems.

"You can get the same effect by taking a traditional NSAID with misoprostol or a similar stomach-protective medication," Dr. Moskowitz explains. "But taking Arthrotec is more convenient, because the drugs have already been combined."

The drawbacks: While Arthrotec is less likely to cause serious gastrointestinal trouble than traditional NSAIDs, it's more likely to cause gassiness and diarrhea, Dr. El-Gabalawy says. Otherwise, the side effects of the two drugs are similar to those of traditional NSAIDs.

It may be right for you if . . . you're at high risk for gastrointestinal problems and you're not getting good results with a COX-2 or meloxicam. Then Arthrotec may be a good choice, Dr. El-Gabalawy says.

It may not be right for you if . . . you're pregnant or trying to get pregnant, since misoprostol can cause miscarriage. Like traditional NSAIDs, Arthrotec may not be appropriate if you have kidney problems, high blood pressure, or heart disease, or if you are allergic to NSAIDs.

For maximum effectiveness: Take with food or milk.

Hyaluronan (Hyalgan), Hylan G-F 20 (Synvisc)

The benefits: Hyaluronan and hylan are viscosupplements, or hyaluronic acid substitutes. They're injected directly into joints, where they fill in for natural hyaluronic acid, a lubricant that breaks down in osteoarthritis.

These medications, which are most effective in

MEDICATIONS WITH MUSCLE

Over-the-counter (OTC) arthritis preparations such as Extra Strength Bayer Arthritis Pain Regimen Formula, Ecotrin Arthritis Relief, and Bufferin Arthritis Strength supply a larger dose of nonsteroidal anti-inflammatory drug (NSAID) than their standard OTC counterparts. The higher the dose, the stronger the pain relief—and the greater the chance of gastrointestinal and other side effects, says Jack Klippel, M.D., medical director of the Atlanta-based Arthritis Foundation.

To offset the risk of gastrointestinal trouble, many of these preparations come with coatings or in time-release formulations. But these special features won't prevent the same sorts of side effects that can occur with other NSAIDs—from ringing in the ears to liver and kidney damage.

---

mild cases of osteoarthritis, can relieve pain for several months, Dr. El-Gabalawy says. They don't work for everyone, but they work extremely well for some, Dr. Klippel adds.

The drawbacks: The injections can cause temporary inflammation, which usually goes away on its own. If it doesn't, you can get a shot of cortisone to clear up the problem. Since the FDA has approved hyaluronic acid substitutes only for osteoarthritis of the knee, insurers usually won't cover treatment of other joints.

They may be right for you if . . . you're not getting relief from traditional NSAIDs, the COX-2s, or meloxicam, and you're not a candidate for surgery. In your case, hyaluronic acid substitutes may be just what you're looking for, Dr. Klippel says.

They may not be right for you if . . . you're allergic to eggs, feathers, or chickens, since hyaluronic acid substitutes are manufactured from rooster and chicken combs.

HELP FOR RHEUMATOID ARTHRITIS

Heidi McIntyre was just 15 years old when she learned she had rheumatoid arthritis (RA). Another 12 years would pass before she got real help for her condition, beyond a doctor's advice to "take some aspirin." By then, she could hardly walk without pain; just getting dressed took time and effort. Eventually, the Atlanta-based McIntyre would require total hip replacement surgery. Her hands are permanently deformed.

For Diana Gru, a teacher in the Philadelphia area, RA came on literally overnight. The pain and inflammation started in her wrists, then jumped to her fingers and toes. She consulted a rheumatologist, who diagnosed RA and prescribed drug therapy right away. After trying several medications, Gru found some that not only alleviated her pain but also slowed the progression of the disease. "I can do everything I used to," she says. That includes exercising—a combination of yoga, step aerobics, treadmill, and stair-climber—and playing the violin.

As these two stories illustrate, the medical approach to RA has changed dramatically over the years. Perhaps the most important development is this: Early diagnosis, followed by early aggressive treatment, can reduce pain, joint damage, and permanent disability—which can help people with RA remain active and independent for a lifetime.

Even for those like McIntyre who have had RA for

years, the news from the pharmaceutical front is better than ever. Since 1998, the FDA has approved four new treatments for RA. More are on the horizon. While none of them is a cure, these drug therapies have profoundly changed the downward course of a once inevitably crippling condition.

For McIntyre, one of the new medications, etanercept (Enbrel), has made a world of difference. In recent years, she has gone on a cruise with her husband and traveled to Disney World with a friend and two young boys. "At one time, I wouldn't have dreamed of traveling like that," she says. "At least not without a wheelchair." Back when McIntyre first found out about her RA, the standard protocol among doctors was to put off prescribing more powerful drugs for as long as possible. This would spare patients the potent side effects, which can include liver damage, kidney damage, and blood problems.

Now, doctors understand that RA can cause permanent disability within a few years or even months. So when they diagnose the condition, they immediately prescribe what are called disease-modifying antirheumatic drugs (DMARDs). This more aggressive treatment has become the gold standard in RA care.

Know Your Options

If you have RA, chances are you're taking at least two different kinds of medication: an NSAID or a corticosteroid, to minimize your symptoms; and a DMARD to slow the progression of the condition before it damages your joints.

While NSAIDs and corticosteroids work fast,

DON'T KEEP YOUR DOCTOR IN THE DARK

In a survey involving 2,248 people, 18 percent reported that they had experienced what they had believed to be side effects of medications. But according to their charts, only 3 percent had actually told their physicians.

"If a drug reaction is causing significant worry, discomfort, or interference with daily activities, contact your physician immediately. Don't be shy," urges Tejal K. Gandhi, M.D., M.P.H., study author and director of patient safety at Brigham and Women's Hospital in Boston. "Changing the dosage or the prescription could help tremendously."

She recommends taking all of your medications, or at least a list of them, to every doctor's visit. Be sure to mention any side effects, as well as any allergic reactions you've noticed. Also share your list with your pharmacist whenever you get a new prescription.

DMARDs sometimes take several weeks to several months to produce results. They do inhibit the advance of RA, but often in exchange for intolerable side effects. None of them appears to produce what rheumatologists and their patients have been searching for: long-term remission.

To address some of these shortcomings, scientists have developed a new generation of DMARDs. They're so different from the originals that they've been given their own classification: biologic response modifiers (BRM), or biologics for short.

The biologics disrupt the inflammation process by blocking the action of certain proteins associated with swelling and joint damage. Unlike most other RA medications, the biologics aren't pills. They are proteins that must be administered by self-injection, like the insulin for diabetes, or by intravenous infusion, which requires a doctor's care.

So which drug therapy makes the most sense for you? It depends a great deal on how severe your RA is and how rapidly it is progressing. You and your doctor also need to consider side effects, cost, and insurance coverage, as well as the effectiveness of any medication you're already on.

The fact is, about two-thirds of people with RA are getting dramatic results from traditional drug therapies. In their case, switching to another medication may not make much sense. But for the remaining one-third who have not responded to other treatments, the DMARDs and biologics may offer a new lease on life.

Methotrexate (Rheumatrex), Sulfasalazine (Azulfidine), Hydroxychloroquine (Plaquenil), Leflunomide (Arava)

The benefits: These DMARDs alleviate pain and aggressively slow the progression of joint damage. Methotrexate and leflunomide inhibit the immune system, which is involved in the inflammatory process.

The drawbacks: DMARDs work slowly, so they don't offer the immediate relief that NSAIDS and corticosteroids do. People who take DMARDs may experience side effects such as hair loss, skin rashes, headaches, and possibly blood and kidney problems.

They may be right for you if . . . your condition is rapidly progressing and you're at risk for permanent disability. Up to two-thirds of people who take DMARDs will show improvement in their RA symptoms.

They may not be right for you if . . . you're at

risk for stomach and kidney problems. You may do better with the biologics.

Etanercept (Enbrel), Infliximab (Remicade), Anakinra (Kineret)

The benefits: These biologics delay joint damage and reduce the symptoms of moderate to severe, active RA. Perhaps the biggest difference between them and other DMARDs is that they cause fewer side effects. That's because they target only the parts of the immune system that contribute to RA symptoms.

"Good evidence suggests that biologic agents are superior to traditional DMARDs in preventing joint damage," Dr. Klippel says. In a study at Johns Hopkins University in Baltimore, the biologic Enbrel stopped disease progression in 72 percent of RA patients who injected the medication twice a week for a year. By comparison, just 60 percent of patients experienced similar improvement when taking pills of the DMARD methotrexate.

Both Enbrel and Remicade, either alone or in combination with methotrexate, appear to work faster and produce better results than methotrexate alone.

The drawbacks: The biologics are expensive; a year's supply can run between $10,000 and $12,000. Medicare pays for Remicade because it requires intravenous infusion at the doctor's office. Enbrel and Kineret are not covered because they're self-injected.

People who use the biologics may experience pain, swelling, and irritation at the site of their injections. Because the drugs inhibit the inflammatory response, some experts are concerned that they may impair a person's ability to fight infection. Questions about their long-term safety and effectiveness remain.

They may be right for you if . . . you haven't seen much improvement with other RA drugs. Because of the high cost of biologics, your doctor may recommend them only if your insurance covers them.

They may not be right for you if . . . they aren't affordable.

CHAPTER FOUR

The Lowdown on Arthritis Supplements

Have you browsed the supplement aisle of your local drugstore or health food store lately? If so, you've probably spotted dozens of products that promise to heal damaged joints and end arthritis pain. And you may have wondered, Do they really work?

In fact, some do live up to their claims. But others aren't worth the plastic they're bottled in. Unfortunately, Americans throw away an estimated $10 billion a year on these unproven and ineffective arthritis formulas.

That's why we've put together this guide: to help sort the legitimate products from the modern-day snake oil. For any supplement not presented here, you can use our seven-point checklist on the opposite page to decide whether it's a good buy.

SHOP SMART

With so many arthritis supplements on the market, you may
not be sure which to buy and which to avoid. This seven-point
checklist can help narrow your choices, so you can make a de-
cision with confidence. But always check with your doctor
before you start supplementing, especially if you're taking any
medication—whether for arthritis or something else.

- [ ] Buy your supplements at stores you trust.
- [ ] Choose products from large companies. They value their
  reputations.
- [ ] Check the product label for the amount of active ingredient.
  It should be there.
- [ ] Avoid products that use words such as "scientific break-
  through" or "miracle cure."
- [ ] Be wary of products that claim to cure all types of arthritis.
- [ ] Bear in mind that natural doesn't necessarily mean safe.
- [ ] Remember: If a product sounds too good to be true, it prob-
  ably is.

WORTH A TRY

All of the following supplements have scientific research and/or anecdotal evidence to support their
claims for arthritis relief and joint health. Of course,
they may not produce the same results for everyone.
You need to experiment to determine which ones
might benefit you. (If you're taking any arthritis medication, talk with your doctor before adding any of
these supplements to your self-care regimen.)

Glucosamine and Chondroitin

The claim: Glucosamine repairs cartilage damage, while chondroitin draws fluid into cartilage to enhance its shock absorption. Combine the two supplements, and you have a promising formula for relieving osteoarthritis symptoms.

The proof: In studies, people with mild to moderate osteoarthritis who took glucosamine and chondroitin reported a level of pain relief similar to that of nonsteroidal anti-inflammatory drugs (NSAIDs) like aspirin and ibuprofen. Research also has shown that the combination of supplements helps slow cartilage damage.

Suggested dosage: 500 milligrams of glucosamine and 400 milligrams of chondroitin, divided into three doses.

Caution: If you are allergic to shellfish, you may experience an adverse reaction to glucosamine. In addition, some studies suggest that glucosamine may aggravate insulin resistance, which means you should monitor your blood sugar while supplementing. The combination of glucosamine and chondroitin may take 8 weeks to produce results.

MSM (Methyl Sulfonyl Methane)

The claim: MSM may alleviate the pain of osteoarthritis by enhancing the effects of cortisol, the body's own anti-inflammatory agent.

The proof: While some anecdotal evidence suggests that MSM may relieve pain, no published studies to date have substantiated the supplement's therapeutic powers. Still, MSM appears to be safe. So if you don't get results from other supplements, this one might merit a trial run.

Suggested dosage: 1,000 milligrams a day.

Caution: Do not use MSM if you are allergic or sensitive to sulfur-containing drugs, or if you take anticoagulants or aspirin on a regular basis. MSM requires at least 4 weeks, if not longer, to work.

SAM-e (S-Adenosylmethionine)

The claim: SAM-e may reduce osteoarthritis pain and improve joint mobility by raising levels of the amino acid ATP and supporting cartilage production.

The proof: Some studies have shown that SAM-e relieves mild osteoarthritis pain almost as well as NSAIDs, but without the gastrointestinal side effects.

Suggested dosage: 200 to 400 milligrams a day, divided into three doses.

Caution: SAM-e may elevate blood levels of homocysteine, a significant risk factor for cardiovascular disease. If you have or are at risk for heart problems, talk with your doctor before supplementing.

Vitamin E

The claim: A potent antioxidant, vitamin E helps protect joints against damage by harmful renegade molecules known as free radicals. It fights pain, swelling, and morning stiffness.

The proof: Some studies have found that vitamin

E is more effective at easing pain than an NSAID or a placebo.

Suggested dosage: 400 IU a day. Because getting this amount from foods is difficult, many experts recommend taking supplements instead.

Caution: If you use anticoagulants or aspirin regularly, consult your doctor before supplementing.

Fish Oil

The claim: The omega-3 fatty acids in fish oil—eicosapentaenoic acid (EPA) and docosahexaenoic acid (DHA)—may fight the pain and stiffness of rheumatoid arthritis by providing the body with anti-inflammatory building blocks.

The proof: In numerous studies, fish oil has proven that it can help relieve the inflammation and accompanying pain of rheumatoid arthritis. It may reduce the need for NSAIDs such as ibuprofen.

Suggested dose: A total of 3,000 milligrams a day from EPA and DHA. If you prefer, you can get these fatty acids from foods—especially cold-water fish such as sardines, salmon, tuna, and mackerel. Aim for 2 or 3 servings a week.

Cautions: Do not use fish oil if you have a bleeding disorder or uncontrolled high blood pressure, if you are taking anticoagulants or aspirin regularly, or if you are allergic to any kind of fish. Also, be sure to get *fish* oil, not *fish-liver* oil, which can contain toxic amounts of vitamins A and D.

GLA (Gamma Linolenic Acid)

The claim: The body converts GLA, an omega-6 fatty acid, into anti-inflammatory compounds.

The proof: Studies have shown that GLA can relieve the inflammation, tenderness, and morning stiffness associated with rheumatoid arthritis. It may reduce the need for NSAIDs such as aspirin, naproxen, and acetaminophen.

Suggested dosage: 1,800 milligrams a day from evening primrose oil, borage oil, or black currant seed oil.

Caution: Consult your doctor before supplementing if you have a seizure disorder or you take aspirin or anticoagulants on a regular basis.

SAVE YOUR MONEY

Because arthritis is so painful and so persistent, some people will try anything—including unproven and sometimes downright harmful products—for relief. Here are a few popular remedies that have not stood up to scientific scrutiny, at least as arthritis treatments. (One or two may be helpful for other conditions.)

Alfalfa: Despite its long history as a folk remedy for arthritis, alfalfa has yet to prove itself in studies.

Copper bracelets: Absolutely no scientific evidence supports the anti-arthritis claims for copper.

DMSO (dimethyl sulfoxide): A by-product of wood processing, DMSO is said to ease pain and improve flexibility in people with arthritis. But many DMSO products currently on the market aren't suit-

STORMY WEATHER, ACHING JOINTS?

Folk wisdom has long contended that people with arthritis can predict the weather. Now science suggests that it may be true.

"It isn't just something people invented," says Robert N. Jamison, Ph.D., director of the pain management program at Brigham and Women's Hospital in Boston and author of *Learning to Master Your Chronic Pain*. "There is a bit of physiological reasoning to support it."

In a four-city survey by Dr. Jamison and his colleagues of 558 people with chronic pain, two-thirds of the respondents said that weather changes affected their symptoms. Of these, a bit more than half reported that their pain worsened even before the weather noticeably shifted.

Curiously, the people living in warm, dry climates actually reported greater sensitivity to weather changes than people living in cold, damp conditions. According to Dr. Jamison, this suggests that barometric pressure is responsible for ratcheting up pain, not temperature or humidity.

Typically, barometric pressure drops before the onset of inclement weather. When the air pressure outside your body falls, the tendons, ligaments, and other tissues surrounding your joints adjust and expand. This squeezes the nerves, which then send pain signals to your brain, Dr. Jamison theorizes.

But if local weather patterns don't agree with your joints, moving may not be the answer. That's because Dr. Jamison and his colleagues also found evidence that the body adjusts to a new climate fairly rapidly.

Suppose you live in Boston and you take a 2-week vacation to San Diego. While there, you might notice a decrease in your pain. But if you moved to San Diego, subtle weather changes—even a modest temperature dip below 70°F—might trigger the same degree of discomfort you thought you had left behind in frigid New England.

If weather changes seem imminent, your best bet may be to pare down your schedule and pace yourself, Dr. Jamison suggests. That way, you'll have plenty of time to rest if your arthritis flares up.

able for humans. They're chemically impure and potentially harmful.

Shark cartilage: Though advertised as a treatment for osteoarthritis and rheumatoid arthritis, shark cartilage has no scientifically acceptable evidence to confirm its therapeutic value. It can cause nausea, vomiting, and fatigue.

CHAPTER FIVE

Nature's Answers to Achy Joints

Sometimes the winds of change can be pretty dramatic. Case in point: A new generation of arthritis drugs is blowing away its predecessors. These days, people can pick and choose from a host of medications proven to ease joint pain and stiffness. And if the latest research is any indication, the number of pharmaceutical options will continue to grow in the years ahead.

Occasionally, though, the winds of change can be subtle. For example, a small but growing group of rheumatologists is quietly transforming the standard treatment protocol for arthritis by routinely recommending a combination of conventional and alternative therapies to their patients. This is a welcome trend for people who want to reduce their dependence on medications, or who have been living with nasty side effects.

In terms of side effects, perhaps the greatest offenders—and certainly one of the most commonly prescribed—are the NSAIDs (short for nonsteroidal anti-inflammatory drugs). While these pills effectively mask pain, they also cause intestinal bleeding, which lands thousands of people in the hospital each year. What's more, laboratory studies suggest that long-term use of NSAIDs actually damages joint tissue.

For those people who don't get good results with NSAIDs, doctors may prescribe corticosteroids. But C. Leigh Broadhurst, Ph.D., a nutrition consultant and herbal researcher based in Clovery, Maryland, contends that treating arthritis with corticosteroids is like cutting down a tree to get rid of a hornet's nest high up in the branches. The pain is gone, but at what price?

Dr. Broadhurst is one of many experts who believe that herbal medicine can control arthritis symptoms with few, if any, side effects. But this particular therapy can be hampered by poor eating habits. So alternative health practitioners recommend a diet of whole grains, fruits, and vegetables—with very little meat, dairy, or refined carbohydrates—to their arthritis patients, says Ruth Bar-Shalom, N.D., a naturopathic physician in Fairbanks, Alaska. She also recommends a daily multivitamin and an antioxidant supplement, which she says can help preserve joint tissue. (To learn more about eating for joint health, see Chapter 7.)

While some herbal remedies target pain, the general objective of herbal medicine is to cleanse the congested tissues surrounding affected joints. Certain herbs stimulate blood flow and digestion and support toxin elimination, which can cause inflammation. In this way, they help stimulate the healing process.

If the therapeutic potential of herbal medicine has piqued your interest, you should consult your doctor or a qualified alternative health practitioner before you begin treatment. Certain herbs might adversely interact with medications you're already taking, making you feel worse instead of better. Be sure to ask about the following remedies, which have the best track records for arthritis relief.

BOSWELLIA

Inside the fragrant frankincense tree are compounds called boswellic acids. Research suggests the acids disrupt inflammation in its earliest stages by inhibiting the production of chemicals that initiate the pain process. In other words, instead of trying to stop a train as it's barreling down the track at 100 miles an hour, boswellia cuts the engines while the train is still pulling out of the station.

The bark of the frankincense tree, which grows on the dry hills of India, supplies the aromatic gum resin used to make a standardized boswellia extract. In studies, the extract has improved blood supply to the joints and prevented the tissue breakdown associated with all kinds of arthritis.

To ease chronic pain, take 450 milligrams of boswellia extract in capsule form four times a day. The herb is safe to use indefinitely, with no apparent side effects.

TURMERIC

Curcumin, the powerful anti-inflammatory compound in turmeric, is not a drug. But it can act like one, Dr.

Broadhurst says. "If my fate were such that I could have only one medicinal plant, I would choose turmeric," she enthuses.

In India, turmeric has a long history of use in medicine, as well as in cooking and dyeing. But it was largely overlooked in the United States until the 1970s, when it was subjected to scientific scrutiny. It certainly held its own. In one clinical study, curcumin proved as effective as the popular anti-inflammatory drug phenylbutazone in treating arthritis symptoms.

To relieve chronic pain and inflammation, take one or two 400- to 500-milligram capsules of turmeric extract three times a day. The herb is safe to use indefinitely.

GINGER

Unlike many arthritis medications that may wreak havoc on your gastrointestinal tract, ginger is a well-known stomach soother. In fact, it's among the most effective remedies—herbal or pharmaceutical—for nausea. Now research suggests that it may work for arthritis, too, Dr. Broadhurst says. In a Danish study, for example, three-quarters of the people with arthritis who took a daily dose of ginger reported reductions in their pain and swelling but no side effects.

You can get relief from your arthritis symptoms by eating about 1 teaspoon of grated ginger every day. For the greatest medicinal potency, choose fresh, organically grown rhizome, sometimes mistakenly referred to as the root. A rhizome that's shriveled, moldy, or chemically treated will not yield as much of the herb's therapeutic compounds.

HEAT FOR THE PAIN

You love the fire of chile peppers in your salsa. But on your skin?

You bet. When applied as a cream, capsaicin—the stuff that puts the heat in chile peppers—can ease the discomfort of arthritis.

Researchers believe that capsaicin works by depleting nerve cells and receptors of substance P, a chemical that transmits pain and itch sensations to the brain. When a capsaicin cream is applied to the skin, the nerves release a flood of substance P. Over time, they can't replenish their supplies of the chemical. The less "fuel" they have, the less pain you feel.

Even though you can buy capsaicin creams over the counter, make no mistake: They're *strong*. So be sure to consult your doctor before buying one, says Rup Tandan, M.D., a neurologist at the University of Vermont in Burlington. Once you have your doctor's okay, follow Dr. Tandan's tips to use the cream safely and effectively.

- Start with a mild formulation. Zostrix has a concentration of 0.025 percent, while Zostrix HP has three times the potency—0.075 percent.
- Apply the cream with a rubber glove or a rubber finger guard. "If you don't and you accidentally put your finger in your eye, it could be bad," Dr. Tandan explains.
- Use a very small amount of cream. "If you can see it on your skin, that's too much," Dr. Tandan says.
- Avoid applying the cream within 2 hours of a hot bath or shower. "Heat increases the cream's effect, which can intensify the pain," Dr. Tandan notes.
- Don't give up. "Your skin may burn for a few days as it adjusts to the cream," Dr. Tandan says. The discomfort will diminish quickly. In most cases, the cream will produce results within about two weeks.

AN ESSENTIAL ARTHRITIS RUB

To soothe arthritic joints, you can make this rub developed by Douglas Schar, a medical herbalist in London, editor of the *British Journal of Phytotherapy*, and author of *Backyard Medicine Chest*. "A medicated rub containing pure essential oils can ease joint pain and inflammation," he explains.

    20 drops lemon essential oil
    20 drops sandalwood essential oil
    I small jar petroleum jelly, minus I tablespoon

Mix the lemon and sandalwood oils into the petroleum jelly. Apply a dab to each sore joint four times a day.

To keep a supply of ginger on hand, peel the rhizome and cut it into thick slices. Place the slices in a clean jar, pour in vodka (as a preservative) to cover, and seal with a lid. You can store the ginger in the refrigerator indefinitely.

JUNIPER

To stimulate blood flow and help cleanse an arthritic joint, Keith Robertson, a member of Britain's National Institute of Medical Herbalists and director of education for the Scottish School of Herbal Medicine in Glasgow, recommends a gentle massage with juniper oil. Made from the berries of the juniper tree, this versatile, woody-scented oil also eases pain and tension.

To use it, mix a few drops of juniper oil with 1 cup of vegetable oil and massage into the affected joint. Repeat three or four times a day for up to 2 weeks, then discontinue treatment.

GUAIACUM

According to Robertson, guaiacum specifically targets the pain and swelling associated with rheumatoid arthritis. It stimulates blood flow to the affected joints and flushes away dead and damaged cells caused by inflammation.

Robertson recommends gently simmering guaiacum to coax out the herb's therapeutic properties, a process called decoction. Add 1 teaspoon of guaiacum wood chips to 1 cup of water and bring to a boil. Simmer for 15 to 20 minutes, then strain. Drink up to 3 cups a day during periods of acute pain and inflammation.

GREEN TEA

Green tea contains polyphenols, compounds proven to relieve the pain of rheumatoid arthritis. In laboratory trials, mice that were given green tea extract had much lower rates of arthritis than mice that were not. Of course, these results need to be confirmed with human studies. But green tea is safe, so trying it certainly won't hurt.

To relieve inflammation, drink 3 to 4 cups of green tea a day. If you prefer the decaffeinated variety, check whether the caffeine has been removed through a process called effervescence. This retains the polyphenols. If the label doesn't mention the processing method, contact the manufacturer. Also, be sure to drink your tea plain, as milk may interfere with the polyphenols' action.

CHAPTER SIX

Home Remedies That Work

Even though arthritis has been around for eons—its telltale signs are etched into fossilized human remains dating back to the Ice Age—it remained largely a mystery until well into the 20th century. It didn't even have a name until the 1800s, let alone an accurate definition. Effective treatments would follow much later.

"Our understanding of arthritis is dramatically better than it was 50 years ago," affirms Ted Fields, M.D., a rheumatologist at the Hospital for Special Surgery in New York City. "And the treatments are dramatically better as well."

As we've seen, the medications to relieve arthritis pain and stiffness continue to multiply. Herbal and nutritional supplements are proving their therapeutic value, too. But they are not your only options. A whole host of self-care strategies can snuff out arthritis symptoms, allowing you to move about with ease and comfort. Here's just a sampling.

Chill out, warm up. Heat, cold, or a combination of the two can provide quick, temporary relief from arthritis pain and stiffness, doctors say. Cold packs numb sore joints and reduce inflammation, while heat therapy stimulates circulation and relaxes muscles.

"In my own experience, I'd say that 60 percent of my patients find 10- to 15-minute applications of moist heat to be most helpful. But the other 40 percent feel that ice is better," Dr. Fields says. "No two people respond the same way to any one treatment. I would recommend using whatever works best for your particular symptoms."

Another option is to try alternating between heat and cold. Dr. Fields suggests applying ice wrapped in a thin towel for 10 minutes. Wait for 10 minutes, then wrap the affected joint in a warm, moist towel for 15 minutes. Repeat as necessary.

Create a diversion from pain. When used as directed, over-the-counter liniments such as Bengay ointment and Icy Hot cream can provide a temporary reprieve from your arthritis symptoms, says Harry Shen, M.D., a rheumatologist at the Hospital for Joint Diseases in New York City.

"Basically, these liniments are counterirritants," Dr. Shen explains. "It's like being at a cocktail party. How many people can you listen to at the same time? One, maybe two. The same principle applies to your body. If you create a sensation of warmth on the skin, it distracts your brain from the painful joint."

Feel soreness wane with wax. For arthritis of the hands, a hot-wax treatment offers soothing relief, says Arnold Katz, M.D., a rheumatologist at the Overland Park Regional Medical Center in Overland Park,

Kansas. You can get the treatment at hospitals and salons, but it's less expensive at home.

Hot-wax (or paraffin) treatment kits are available in medical supply stores as well as some pharmacies and department stores. Be sure to read and follow the instructions for the kit you purchase. Most work about the same: You warm the wax in a heating unit and apply it to your hands. Leave on the wax for 10 minutes, wearing a pair of plastic gloves while you wait.

The beauty of an in-home hot-wax treatment is that you can reuse the wax for several weeks. Just be careful if you have youngsters in your home, Dr. Katz cautions. They could knock over the heating unit and burn themselves.

Pick a point and press. Acupressure, which involves applying pressure to specific points on the body—the same points used in acupuncture—can quickly squash arthritis symptoms, says Dharma Singh Khalsa, M.D., a pain management expert in Tucson, Arizona, and author of *The Pain Cure*. It works by signaling the brain to release endorphins, natural opiates that reduce the perception of pain.

Although acupressure's effects are only temporary—lasting from 15 to 20 minutes—it can come in handy at those times when longer-lasting relief isn't readily available, Dr. Khalsa says. To try it, simply apply pressure to whichever of the following points corresponds to your aching joint. Keep pressing until the pain dissipates, which could take from 3 to 5 minutes.

- For arthritis of the fingers and wrist, press on the hollow on the back of your wrist, in line with your index finger.

- For arthritis of the wrist or hand, press at the top of the webbing between your thumb and index finger.
- For arthritis of the shoulder, press on the inside of your elbow, on the same side as your thumb.
- For arthritis of the knee, press in the hollow beneath your kneecap.

You can tell if you're in the right spot because acupressure points are more sensitive than the surrounding areas. You need to press hard enough that your brain senses it and releases endorphins in response.

Request a rubdown. Massage helps relieve arthritis pain by pushing blood and other bodily fluids through the bloodstream, which reduces swelling and eliminates waste products from tissues. Many health clubs and day spas have licensed massage therapists on staff. If that isn't in your budget, you can always recruit your spouse or a friend to give you a soothing 10-minute massage.

Immobilize the aching joint. Wearing a splint, a sling, or a similar device can protect an arthritic joint against bumps and movement, says David Richards, M.D., an orthopedic surgeon at the Lexington Clinic Sports Medicine Center in Lexington, Kentucky. The catch is, you need to limit your use of such a device to a couple of days at most. Any longer, and it could weaken your muscles. Besides, if an arthritis flare-up lasts longer than a day or two, you should see your doctor anyway.

Kick off those heels. If you're a woman with a

PAIN ON PINS AND NEEDLES

Other alternative healing disciplines may be less invasive. But acupuncture has one mighty advantage: It's swift.

"It is one of the fastest-acting natural arthritis pain relievers available," says Patrick LaRiccia, M.D., a physician and registered acupuncturist who works as director of the Acupuncture Pain Clinic at Presbyterian Medical Center of Philadelphia. "And it certainly is a very powerful one—more powerful than a TENS (transcutaneous electrical nerve stimulation) unit or a hot compress. In a group of 100 people with painful joints, I'd expect acupuncture to provide relief for at least 80 percent of them."

Acupuncture works by stimulating the production of natural painkilling hormones called endorphins, as well as the anti-inflammatory hormone adrenocorticotropin. Inserting needles into the skin at certain points on the body reduces the muscle spasms, inflammation, and pain associated with arthritis, Dr. LaRiccia explains. In addition, it helps increase the range of motion in stiff joints.

Early research appears to confirm acupuncture's effectiveness in alleviating arthritis symptoms. In a pilot study at the University of Maryland in Adelphi, 12 people with osteoarthritis reported improvement in their symptoms after receiving acupuncture treatment. In his own small study, Dr. LaRiccia found that acupuncture alters activity in the areas of the brain that perceive pain.

While more research is necessary, these findings are significant. As Dr. LaRiccia notes, "Acupuncture has a clear physiological effect. People are not just imagining it. Something really is going on."

fondness for high heels, be aware that they can aggravate arthritis symptoms, says Andrew T. Weil, M.D., director of the program in integrative medicine at the University of Arizona College of Medicine in

Tucson. In fact, women are twice as likely as men to develop osteoarthritis of the knees, and heels may be partly responsible for that.

For a study at Harvard Medical School and Spaulding Hospital, both in Boston, researchers recruited 20 healthy women who habitually wore heels at least 2 inches high. The women were asked to walk at a comfortable pace both barefoot and in their shoes. Using video cameras and sensors, the researchers determined that walking in high heels increased the strain on the insides of the knees—the areas most prone to arthritic degeneration—by 23 percent.

At this point, no one knows the exact heel height that begins to raise the risk of arthritis. But wearing flats probably is a whole lot healthier than stressing your knees in heels, Dr. Weil says.

Exercise your funny bone. Laughter is a powerful weapon against pain, says Robert N. Jamison, Ph.D., director of the pain management program at Brigham and Women's Hospital in Boston and author of *Learning to Master Your Chronic Pain*. It relaxes tense muscles, distracts your mind, and decreases the production of stress-related hormones.

"Pain is terribly serious, and it causes such misery that distancing yourself from it is hard," Dr. Jamison explains. "But laughter can renew your sense of why life is worth living. Any means of finding humor in your existence can help."

So if you're having a particularly rough day, imagine how your favorite comedian might describe it. Then you may be able to laugh it off. Reserve a space on your refrigerator or bulletin board for cartoons and funny pictures or sayings that can evoke a chuckle just when you need one. Create a library of humorous writings and videos that can provide comic relief during an arthritis flare-up. Do whatever lightens your mood and alleviates your symptoms. After all, laughter *is* the best medicine.

PART III

Living Arthritis-Free

CHAPTER SEVEN

Eating to End Pain

Want to try a traditional Chinese remedy for arthritis? Combine 100 dead snakes with 5 liters of red wine and some herbs. Let mellow for three months. Then drink the wine three times a day for 6 to 12 weeks.

Admittedly, this concoction is a bit on the strange side. But until recently, many in the medical establishment viewed any food-related remedy for arthritis as only slightly less bizarre than this unappetizing brew.

While no specific food can cure osteoarthritis or rheumatoid arthritis, doctors today recognize that what people eat—and, in some cases, don't eat—can help ease symptoms and possibly slow the progression of the disease. In this chapter, we'll review some of the basic dietary guidelines for maintaining healthy joints. (For an easy-to-follow menu plan and more than 30 healing recipes, see Part IV.)

VITAMIN C DERAILS DAMAGE

Of all the different kinds of arthritis, osteoarthritis might seem the least likely to have some sort of dietary connection. After all, it is a "natural" result of wear and tear in the joints. Can a person's eating habits really have an impact?

Apparently, they can—at least according to a preliminary study at Boston University School of Medicine. Researchers there studied the diets of people who had osteoarthritis of the knee. Those who got the most vitamin C (more than 200 milligrams a day) were three times less likely to experience progression of the disease than those who got the least vitamin C (less than 120 milligrams a day).

The researchers aren't certain why vitamin C intake made such a difference, says study leader Timothy McAlindon, M.D., assistant professor of medicine. Since vitamin C is an antioxidant, it may protect joints from the damaging effects of free radicals—unstable oxygen molecules that can cause joint inflammation. "Vitamin C also may help generate collagen, which enhances the body's ability to repair damage to the cartilage," Dr. McAlindon says.

He advises people with osteoarthritis to get at least 120 milligrams of vitamin C a day, twice the Daily Value. "That's the amount in a couple of oranges," he notes. Other good sources include cantaloupe, broccoli, strawberries, peppers, and cranberry juice.

FISHING FOR RELIEF

High fat intake can contribute to a number of conditions, including arthritis (more on this later in the chapter). But one particular kind of fat actually can help arthritic joints. The omega-3 fatty acids, found primarily in cold-water fish, reduce the body's production of prostaglandins and leukotrienes. Both of these substances contribute to inflammation.

For a study at Albany Medical College in New York, researchers instructed 37 people with arthritis to consume large amounts of fish oil, which supplies omega-3's. After six months, these people reported fewer tender joints, less morning stiffness, and better grip strength than a group that consumed less or no fish oil.

While scientific studies often require the use of supplements, you can get your omega-3's by eating fish, according to a study at the University of Washington in Seattle. Researchers there found that women who ate at least one serving of baked or broiled fish a week were less likely to develop rheumatoid arthritis than women who didn't.

To get the full therapeutic benefit of fish, you should eat two or three servings a week, says Joanne Curran-Celentano, R.D., Ph.D., associate professor of nutritional sciences at the University of New Hampshire in Durham. For omega-3's, your best bets include salmon, bluefin tuna, rainbow trout, halibut, and pollack, as well as canned fish such as mackerel, herring, and sardines.

LESS FAT, HEALTHIER JOINTS

The omega-3s are among a group of "good fats" that
promote optimum health in a variety of ways. In general, though, a diet low in fat—especially saturated
fat—appears to be the smartest choice for controlling
arthritis symptoms.

In one study, 23 people with rheumatoid arthritis
followed a very low fat diet (supplying just 10 percent
of calories as fat) for 12 weeks. They also walked for
30 minutes a day and took steps to rein in stress. Over
the course of the study, these people experienced a 20
to 40 percent reduction in joint tenderness and swelling. Many were able to cut back on their arthritis medications. By comparison, a second group that didn't
follow a very low fat diet showed no improvement in
their symptoms. The researchers attributed the different outcomes in the two groups to fat intake.

A diet low in saturated fat slows the body's production of inflammatory prostaglandins, says study
leader Edwin H. Krick, M.D., associate professor of
medicine at Loma Linda University in California.
What's more, it may hinder communications from the
immune system, effectively interrupting the inflammatory response. This gives joints a chance to heal,
Dr. Krick explains.

Some doctors recommend limiting dietary fat to no
more than 25 percent of total calories, with no more
than 7 percent of those calories coming from saturated
fat. "One very simple way to cut back on saturated
fat is to not add it to food," says David Pisetsky,
M.D., Ph.D., co-director of the Duke University Ar-

thritis Center in Durham, North Carolina, and medical adviser to the Arthritis Foundation. "For example, when you have a sandwich, use low-fat mayonnaise instead of the real thing."

Replacing full-fat butter, sour cream, and cheese with low-fat or fat-free varieties also helps lower your saturated fat intake. Even if you don't completely eliminate it from your diet, just cutting back can make a difference.

THE ADVANTAGE OF VEGETARIANISM

Besides being a primary source of saturated fat in the standard American diet, meat contains proteins that may play a role in arthritis pain. So in theory, going vegetarian could help aching joints. Research seems to bear this out.

In a study at the University of Oslo in Norway, 27 people with rheumatoid arthritis followed a vegetarian diet for one year. After the first 3 to 5 months, they could eat dairy products, if they wished. But they avoided gluten (a protein found in wheat), refined sugar, salt, alcohol, and caffeine for the duration. After just one month, they reported less swelling and tenderness in their joints. They also had less morning stiffness and stronger grips than people who stayed with their usual diets.

"In populations with diets of mostly unprocessed fruits, vegetables, and grains, autoimmune diseases like rheumatoid arthritis are almost nonexistent," notes Joel Fuhrman, M.D., a specialist in nutritional medicine at the Amwell Health Center in Belle Mead, New Jersey. "You don't see much crippling rheumatoid arthritis in rural China, for example, because the people there eat differently than we Americans do."

FOODS THAT TRIGGER FLARE-UPS

Since rheumatoid arthritis results from an overzealous immune system, and since immune function depends to some degree on diet, what people eat very well may influence how their joints feel—for better or for worse.

Some people are sensitive to certain foods, like wheat, dairy, corn, citrus fruits, tomatoes, and eggs. These can switch on the body's inflammatory response, setting the stage for a rheumatoid arthritis flare-up.

But foods may not be the only culprit. In a recent study involving more than 30,000 men and women, those who drank decaffeinated coffee were twice as likely to develop rheumatoid arthritis as those who drank regular coffee and tea. "We don't yet know what's behind this phenomenon, but it may have something to do with how decaffeinated coffee is processed or brewed," says study author Ted Mikuls, M.D., of the University of Alabama at Birmingham.

Because so many things can aggravate rheumatoid arthritis, determining which (if any) foods you should avoid can be difficult. Dr. Pisetsky suggests keeping a food diary, so you can see what you're eating when your flare-ups occur. If you discover a pattern—for example, your joints ache whenever you eat tomatoes or tomato-based products—eliminate that food from your diet for at least 5 days, he says. Then try it again.

PAINT THE TOWN RED . . . WITH CHERRIES

Folklore is full of stories about people who relieved the agonizing pain of gout by eating cherries or drinking cherry juice every day. Tart cherries contain antioxidants, nutrients that neutralize free radicals. Damage from these renegade oxygen molecules contributes to a host of ailments, possibly including gout.

While the Arthritis Foundation hasn't found any scientific evidence to confirm the therapeutic power of cherries, many gout sufferers swear by them. In a *Prevention* magazine survey, 67 percent of readers who tried cherries for gout reported good results.

Steve Schumacher, a kinesiologist in Louisville, Kentucky, is a big fan of cherries, too. He advises people with gout to drink two or three glasses of cherry juice a day, in addition to abstaining from red meats and organ meats. He favors pure black-cherry juice diluted with an equal amount of water. "Those who faithfully follow these recommendations have gotten good results—some within 48 to 72 hours and others within a week, depending on the severity of their symptoms," Schumacher says.

If your symptoms return, you probably are sensitive to that food, and you may need to give it up for good.

FASTING MAY SLOW RA SYMPTOMS

Although many doctors aren't convinced that fasting has an effect on rheumatoid arthritis, Dr. Fuhrman believes that it can provide relief. "Virtually everyone with rheumatoid arthritis who goes on a fast finds that their pain goes away, at least temporarily," he says.

In some cases of rheumatoid arthritis, Dr. Fuhrman explains, the immune system works overtime attacking partially digested food particles that escape from the intestines into the bloodstream. Fasting allows the

immune system, and the rest of the body, to recover
from this process. And once you break the fast, you
can reintroduce foods one at a time to determine
which ones are most likely to trigger flare-ups.

For people who don't like the idea of total depri-
vation—even for a day or two—drinking fruit juices,
vegetable juices, and herbal teas is acceptable. This
modified fast can help relieve arthritis pain, while providing the body with essential nutrients.

In general, someone who is healthy can fast for up
to two days without a problem. On the other hand,
this therapy may not be appropriate for people who
have certain medical conditions or who are taking
medication or insulin for diabetes. Be sure to consult
your doctor before you try it.

CHAPTER EIGHT

Keep Those Joints Jumpin'

If you've ever kept a sponge by your kitchen sink, you know what happens when you don't use it very much. Without water, it keeps getting drier and drier until eventually, it can't do its job anymore.

That's kind of what happens to your joints when they remain inactive for too long.

"The saying 'Use it or lose it' is quite fitting for arthritis," says Ted Fields, M.D., a rheumatologist at the Hospital for Special Surgery in New York City. "If you give in to stiffness and pain, if you avoid bending your joints, over time they'll develop scar tissue that makes movement even more difficult and uncomfortable."

On the other hand, regular exercise not only relieves pain and stiffness, it could help reverse arthritis, says Dharma Singh Khalsa, M.D., a pain management expert in Tucson, Arizona, and author of *The Pain Cure*. Among its many benefits, exercise:

Increases the flow of synovial fluid into and

out of joints. Synovial fluid helps nourish and moisten cartilage, so it doesn't deteriorate.

Strengthens muscles, tendons, and ligaments. Strong muscles and supporting tissues help counteract stress and strain on your joints.

Improves the flow of blood. Good circulation delivers nutrients and oxygen to your joints while flushing out toxins and other waste that can aggravate arthritis.

Preserves bone. Exercise supports the absorption of mineral into bones, so they're far more resistant to arthritis.

Controls weight. Excessive weight aggravates arthritic joints.

In addition, exercise increases the production of three potent pain-fighting chemicals: endorphins, serotonin, and norepinephrine. With more of these natural pain relievers in your body, you won't mind your arthritis symptoms as much, Dr. Khalsa says. And you'll feel more able to try other strategies that can help reduce pain and stiffness.

YES, YOU *CAN* EXERCISE!

Both the Arthritis Foundation and many physicians recommend a fitness routine that combines simple range-of-motion exercises—such as bending, reaching, and stretching—with strength-building techniques. Any of the following activities can provide a gentle, low-sweat workout that's good for your joints. (For a more detailed fitness routine, including strength-training and stretching exercises, see Chapter 10.)

TUNE OUT PAINFUL JOINTS

If you struggle to muster the motivation to get through a work-out, try doing your exercises while plugged in to your favorite CD. Listening to music just might provide the nudge you need, at least according to some preliminary research.

In a small study at Glasgow University in Scotland, research-ers found that women with rheumatoid arthritis could walk 30 percent farther when they listened to the music of their choice compared with when they were without tunes. "The music did not alleviate their pain," explains lead researcher Paul Mac-Intyre, M.D. "But it did take their minds off their pain, so they could go longer without needing to stop."

Lace up your walking shoes. Walking is the simplest, least-expensive activity for keeping joints flexible and pain-free. According to the Arthritis Foundation, you should aim for 20 to 30 minutes of walking 3 to 5 days each week. You can do the 20 to 30 minutes all at once or as several short jaunts spread over the course of a day.

Try to plan your walking for when you feel your best—perhaps in the morning because you're more energized, or in the afternoon because you're less stiff. Choose a route that is on flat ground, and wear shoes that are adequately cushioned. Perhaps most important, remember to stretch your muscles afterward.

Act like a clown. Pierre-Auguste Renoir, the famous Impressionist painter, juggled balls for 10 minutes every morning to relieve his rheumatoid arthritis. Maybe you should, too, says David Bilstrom, M.D., director of the physiatric medical acupuncture program at Christ Hospital and Medical Center in Oak Lawn, Illinois.

"Juggling is good exercise for the hands, elbows, and shoulders," Dr. Bilstrom notes. "So it not only improves flexibility, it also helps maintain fine muscle coordination."

If you struggle with juggling, simply tossing and catching a beanbag or a small, lightweight rubber ball for 5 minutes twice a day can help limber up stiff joints. Likewise, knitting or playing a musical instrument such as a recorder is great for stiff fingers, says Michael Loes, M.D., director of the Arizona Pain Institute and coauthor of *Arthritis: The Doctors' Cure*.

Strike up the band. Vigorously conducting a recorded orchestra in the comfort of your home is an excellent technique for loosening arthritic joints, says Kathleen Ferrell, P.T., a physical therapist and associate director of the Washington University Regional Arthritis Center in St. Louis. It provides a terrific aerobic workout to boot. "You don't need to go out. You don't need to change your clothes. You don't need special shoes," Ferrell notes. "If you feel wobbly, you can do it sitting in a chair."

Make a splash. Aquatic exercise can be very kind to your joints, Dr. Bilstrom says. Because of the water's buoyancy, you can move your body with less stress and discomfort. Simply walking in water for 20 minutes 3 days a week provides a good workout for your knees, hips, and lower back. And if you pump your arms as you walk, you'll benefit your upper-body joints as well. You can modify the intensity of your workout by exercising in various depths of water. Start at 3 feet, and as you grow stronger, gradually advance to chest-deep.

Actually, you can get relief without even climbing

FOR GOLFERS: A FAIRWAY SURVIVAL GUIDE

If you love playing golf, don't let arthritis interfere with your game. The Arthritis Foundation offers these tips to stay limber on the links.

☐ Before you tee off, walk for a few minutes to loosen your joints.

☐ Devote 5 to 10 minutes to gentle stretching exercises like trunk twists and hamstring stretches.

☐ Be sure to spend some time on the practice range. Warm up your muscles with a few dozen swings.

If your playing partners aren't sticklers for rules, these strategies can help make for a pain-free round (though they won't guarantee a low score!).

☐ Use a tee for every shot, even on the fairway. You're less likely to strike the ground with your club, which can jar your joints.

☐ If you feel tired, skip the tee area and begin your pursuit of the hole from the 150-yard marker on the fairway.

all the way into the pool. Just sit on the edge and dangle your legs up to midcalf, suggests Jane Katz, Ed.D., professor of health and physical education at the City University of New York, world Masters champion swimmer, and member of the 1964 U.S. Olympic performance synchronized swimming team. First make circles with your feet, rotating your ankles clockwise and then counterclockwise. Next, move your feet forward, back, left, and right, keeping your legs slightly bent and your ankles loose. Repeat each exercise five times.

REMEDIES FOR POST-WORKOUT SORENESS

None of the above activities should aggravate arthritic joints. If you experience severe pain during a workout, stop immediately. You may have a problem other than arthritis that requires prompt medical attention.

For run-of-the-mill soreness after exercising, you can use one of the following remedies for relief. (For additional suggestions, see Chapter 6.) Your discomfort should subside in a day or two, even without treatment. If it doesn't, see your doctor.

Treat with a towel. Moist heat improves blood flow and relaxes tight muscles around joints, according to Dan Hamner, M.D., a physiatrist and sports medicine specialist in New York City. The next time your knee throbs or your elbow swells, wet a hand towel and then put it in the dryer at a high temperature for about 10 minutes. While it's still wet and hot, drape it over your joint, covering it with a dry towel to hold in the heat. Leave it on for about 15 minutes, repeating as necessary for relief.

Give peas a chance. For reducing swelling and inflammation, cold treatments work better than heat. A bag of frozen peas makes an excellent ice pack, since it conforms to the shape of your joint. Wrap the bag in a thin towel and apply it to the affected joint for up to 10 minutes at a time.

Hit the showers. If your neck or back feels stiff, try standing in a hot shower for 10 minutes, advises Jane Sullivan-Durand, M.D., a behavioral medicine physician from Contoocook, New Hampshire. The water should be as hot as you can stand. Allow it to bead on the affected area.

CHAPTER NINE

Mental Medicine for Relief

The relationship between a person's mental and emotional state and physical health remains something of a mystery. But scientists have no doubt that such a relationship exists. Already a volume of impressive research suggests that a positive mindset can enhance the therapeutic powers of diet and exercise, and can help fight a whole host of ailments—including arthritis.

Ironically, several of the healing disciplines that have played prominent roles in the relatively new field of mind-body medicine date back hundreds of years. Today, they're proving their effectiveness in study after study.

So let's travel the bridge between mind and body to explore four distinct therapies with remarkable potential for healing arthritic joints.

IMAGERY

What It Is

The bowler, cursed by spares, envisions the 10 tooth-white pins crumbling in the thunder of a strike. The hockey goalie sees his glove snatching the icy, spinning black puck hurtling toward the net. Just before stepping into the batter's box, the slugger pictures the baseball soaring high over the centerfield wall.

These athletes *will* themselves into action, using their minds in concert with their muscles through a mental technique known as imagery. They've trained their brains to picture their strengths and their successes ahead of time. This ability to imagine good results subdues their worry and anxiety, doctors say.

What works for the stars of the sports world can work for the rest of us. Our minds can convince our bodies to function at their best, even when they're dealing with a condition like arthritis.

Now, the mind is not all-powerful. You can't just think your way to a cure. But research has shown that once you master imagery, you can use it to support and facilitate the healing process.

When you practice imagery, you do more than create a picture in your mind, notes Martin Rossman, M.D., clinical associate in the department of medicine at the University of California Medical Center in San Francisco and codirector of the Academy for Guided Imagery in Mill Valley, California. You engage all five of your senses. Invoking sounds, smells, textures, and tastes helps to enhance the therapeutic benefits.

Imagery works best when it is customized to each individual, says Belleruth Naparstek, a lecturer and expert on guided imagery from Cleveland Heights, Ohio. An image that works for one person may not work for another. Still, virtually anyone can move toward a mental state that's more conducive to physical healing by tapping their ability to vividly imagine things.

"Everybody has an imagination," Naparstek says. "What imagery does is enable us to transcend the limitations of how we see ourselves so that we can access the healing power within ourselves."

What It Does

Imagery is a pain-free technique that has been proven to help arthritis, along with many other health problems. For starters, it's an effective pain reliever. What's more, it can influence body temperature, heart rate, blood pressure, oxygen consumption, gastrointestinal activity, sexual arousal, muscle relaxation, and immune function. "If a pill could stimulate the immune system as the imagination does, it would be a required treatment for immuno-compromised patients," Dr. Rossman says.

Then, too, our ability to marshal our imaginations can effectively counteract stress. It works by reducing levels of stress hormones like adrenaline and cortisol while increasing levels of natural tranquilizers like endorphins. This explains why imagery is especially useful in managing conditions that are caused or complicated by stress.

In a controlled study at the Cleveland Clinic Foundation involving patients undergoing colorectal surgery, those who listened to Naparstek's guided imagery audiotapes before and after their procedures experienced less anxiety beforehand and required less medication afterward. They also were released from the hospital sooner.

Dr. Rossman offers this persuasive example of imagery's power: If you ask someone to salivate, she may or may not to be able to do it. But if you ask the person to close her eyes, take deep, regular breaths, and imagine sucking on a juicy, sour lemon, she probably will salivate—the result of imagery triggering a physiological response.

Start Something!

Now that you're familiar with the principles of imagery, use these strategies to make the most of it in your arthritis management plan.

Practice, practice, practice. Not everyone can master imagery on the first attempt at it. But most get better with practice, Naparstek says.

Train with an expert. For newcomers to imagery, both Naparstek and Dr. Rossman recommend a session or two with a qualified therapist. You want someone who offers suggestions rather than someone who delivers commands to conjure specific images. Envisioning a hike along a pristine mountain trail might seem helpful to the therapist, but it won't work for you if it triggers thoughts of stiff, painful knees.

Talk to your pain. For achy joints, imagery experts suggest creating a picture of your pain and having a mental conversation with it: Why are you here? What do you want? What will convince you to go away? This technique can make the pain seem less intimidating, which in turn may help control it more effectively, Naparstek says.

Smile your way to relief. You might try "disguising" your pain by seeing it as your favorite cartoon character or in a chicken suit. Then you can laugh at it, which will trigger the release of natural painkillers called endorphins. It also will relax tense muscles and loosen tight joints.

Turn your visions into sweet dreams. What if you fall asleep during an imagery session? Don't worry about it, Naparstek says. The therapeutic power of imagery will continue working even after you've nodded off. In fact, it may work even better for some Type A personalities who have trouble relaxing when they're awake, Naparstek notes.

Get in the habit of imagining. Through imagery, you can go anywhere your mind wants. Think of it as a mental mini-vacation. And just as on a "real" vacation, your body can relax and unwind. Of course, your best bet for maximizing these benefits is to use imagery on a daily basis.

Pair it with the practical. Imagery can be a valuable component of your arthritis management plan. But as Dr. Rossman advises, it should not replace medications or other treatments recommended by your doctor. You may still need to take a COX-2 inhibitor to reduce inflammation, for example.

Trial Run

Imagery works best when you close your eyes and envision a place where you feel relaxed and comfort-

THE FAITH FACTOR

A growing body of scientific research appears to affirm the connection between faith and health. One of the most intriguing studies to date comes from Duke University. Though quite small in scale, it offers convincing proof that spiritual beliefs and practices may help people with rheumatoid arthritis cope better with their pain.

Every day for a month, the 35 study participants—all of whom had rheumatoid arthritis—kept specially designed diaries with questionnaires to rate their religion-based coping strategies, pain, mood, and social support. The people who most strongly believed in the effectiveness of religion-based coping strategies had less pain, better moods, and more social support. Their diaries also revealed the following:

Faith needn't be "formal." The study participants were more likely to say that they were touched by the beauty of creation; that they desired to be closer to or in union with God; or that they felt God's love directly or through others.

Positive faith works better. Those who looked to God for strength, support, and guidance fared better than those who wondered whether their illness was a sign that God was punishing them or had abandoned them.

Faith improves personal relationships. The people who reported more frequent spiritual experiences also perceived more social support in their lives.

The Duke study is among the first to evaluate the immediate effects of everyday spiritual experiences on the ability to cope with chronic conditions like rheumatoid arthritis. Further research will confirm the significance of the findings.

able. The trick is to concentrate and involve all of your senses. Relying on your mind's eye isn't enough. You've got to engage your mind's ear and nose, too. That's when imagery can provide a healthy escape from the distractions of pain and inflammation.

As mentioned earlier, if you're trying imagery for the first time, you may benefit from a session or two with a therapist who can provide training in the basic technique. But you're welcome to try it on your own. Here's a sample exercise that Naparstek recommends.

1. To start, think about a time in your life when you felt vibrant and peaceful. Perhaps you were vacationing at the beach with your family, or enjoying dinner with a close friend, or puttering in the garden by yourself. Whatever memory you come up with, make sure it's a positive one.

2. Next, sit in a comfortable chair, rest your hands in your lap, and close your eyes. Inhale deeply, all the way down to your belly. Then exhale as fully and completely as you can.

3. Now, focus on the memory you chose in step 1. As you drift back to that moment in time, reconnect with your feelings and engage all of your senses. If you're remembering a vacation at the beach, for example, try to hear the sound of the waves whooshing onto the sand and then retreating. Smell the brine and sunscreen. Feel the texture of the warm sand. Taste the saltwater on your lips.

4. As you recall all the details, immerse yourself in your memory, until you feel as though you're actually reliving it. You can stay in it for as long as you like. Try for 10 minutes, at least.

5. When you're ready, open your eyes slowly. Allow yourself a minute or so to readjust to the present. Feel your breath filling your lungs.

> Be aware of your feet on the floor, your but-
> tocks on the chair, and your hands in your lap.
> You should feel relaxed and refreshed.

Practice this exercise once a day—more often, if you
can spare the time. By concentrating on a positive,
pleasurable memory, you release the stress and tension that can inhibit your body's ability to heal itself.

MEDITATION

What It Is

While meditation has grown in popularity, it still is
misunderstood by the general public. Many people
think it involves going into a trance, or "zoning out."
In fact, it's the exact opposite.

Meditation is the art of turning inward, of controlling our thought processes. Too often our thoughts
drift around our minds like a bottle in the surf. Meditation stops the drifting by focusing our awareness.

The most serious devotees may practice meditation
while seated either on a cushion on the floor or in a
chair. But you needn't be so formal about it. You can
achieve a meditative state just about anytime and anywhere, even while you're in motion.

In short, meditation is not mystical or magical. It's
a time-tested discipline with proven therapeutic powers, particularly for conditions like arthritis.

What It Does

By influencing your thought patterns, meditation can
improve your ability to cope with arthritis symptoms.

Some experts believe it's so effective that it actually can reduce the frequency of rheumatoid arthritis flare-ups. Other benefits include the following:

Relieves chronic pain. Meditation brings about deep relaxation. As it loosens your muscles and joints, you feel less pain.

Reverses the effects of stress. Meditation reduces levels of harmful stress hormones, which can aggravate arthritis symptoms. In a study at the Center for Health and Aging Studies of the Maharishi University of Management in Fairfield, Iowa, meditators showed an impressive, healthful decline in one particular kind of stress hormone after only 4 months of regular practice. Meditation also can help treat any condition for which stress is a cause or a contributing factor.

Lowers blood pressure. For people with high blood pressure, meditation can be very potent medicine. In one study, it significantly reduced blood pressure readings in just 3 months of daily practice.

Controls nervous system disorders. According to Janet Messer, Ph.D., a psychologist in private practice in Eugene, Oregon, regular meditation seems to counteract certain tic disorders. These disorders produce muscle contractions that lead to facial twitches and other characteristic symptoms like the compulsive explosion of inappropriate words (as in Tourette's syndrome). Although meditation will not cure these symptoms, it can stop them for several hours.

Helps break bad habits. Meditation bestows benefits on the mind as well as the body. In a case study in the department of psychology at Pepperdine University in Culver City, California, researchers found that meditation could help end chronic nervous behaviors such as nail biting.

Develop a healthy self-awareness. Over time, meditation improves your ability to observe your thoughts without reacting to them, even as you're going about your daily routine. You may find that you feel calmer, and that you're less likely to get upset over life's minor annoyances.

Start Something!

The beauty of meditation is that it's so adaptable. Actually, almost any activity that's performed with awareness takes on a meditative quality. For example:

Find delight in dishwashing. For centuries, monks have found serenity in the quiet obligations of labor. So when you see a pile of dirty dishes in the kitchen sink, consider it an opportunity to meditate. As you soap and rinse, don't mentally review the events of the past day or plan your schedule for tomorrow. Instead, stay entirely in the moment. In this way, a task as routine as dishwashing can become quite relaxing, says Mark Epstein, M.D., clinical assistant professor of psychology at New York University and author of *Thoughts without a Thinker* and *Going to Pieces without Falling Apart*.

Focus on your fitness routine. Instead of using your workout sessions to mentally rehash your troubles and worries, tune your attention to your body's movements. You might concentrate on the rhythm of your feet hitting the pavement, or the stroke of each arm pulling through the water, or the air entering and leaving your lungs. "You're putting your mental energy into your physical activity," Dr. Epstein explains. This may be how meditation enhances athletic performance.

Be mindful at mealtime. Even eating can be a meditative experience. And it starts before you take a single bite of food. As you sit down at the table, focus on your breathing until you feel quiet and calm. Then you can pick up your utensils and begin eating. Chew and swallow slowly, concentrating on every bite. Engage your senses by savoring the colors, aromas, and textures of your food. This practice can make your meals more relaxing and pleasurable.

Trial Run

For a more traditional meditation session, you'll want to sit in a chair or cross-legged on a cushion. Relax your shoulders and place your hands in your lap while holding your head, neck, and spine as straight as possible. Close your eyes or lower your eyelids just enough to limit visual distractions. Let your body become still and your mind clear.

The following techniques can help maintain your concentration during your meditation sessions. You may want to try all of them before choosing one that you're comfortable with, Dr. Epstein says.

Be aware of your breath. Buddha, perhaps the most famous meditator of all time, is said to have used this technique to reach the ultimate state of awareness known as enlightenment. For the rest of us, it's one of the simplest methods for achieving deep relaxation and concentration.

To start, focus on your breath, paying attention to each inhalation and exhalation. You may want to direct your mental energy to your belly as it rises and falls, or to your nostrils as the air gently flows in and out.

Don't alter your breathing pattern; just tune in to it. If your mind wanders, refocus on your breath. For this moment, you want your breath to be the most important thing in the world.

Count for clarity. If you're a beginning meditator, you can use counting to facilitate focusing on your breath. Count on either the inhalation or the exhalation, paying attention to both the numbers and your breath. When you reach 10, start over.

Meld with a mantra. Say "meditation," and many people conjure a mental image of a grizzled old swami sitting cross-legged and chanting the same word over and over again. Using words or sounds as mantras—tools for maintaining concentration—is a common practice in many religions, including Christianity and Hinduism. The mantras themselves may vary, but their effects are quite similar. They keep your mind from wandering back to everyday concerns, like mortgage payments and work deadlines and car breakdowns.

Coming up with your own mantra is easy. Just choose a word, a phrase, or a sound that holds a special, positive meaning for you. *Peace*, *love*, *amen*, and *om* are a few examples—but the possibilities are endless!

Once you've decided on a mantra, repeat it to yourself while you meditate. Focus on it just as you would focus on your breath. When other thoughts attempt to intrude—and they will—let your mantra fill your mind instead. With time and practice, you'll experience fewer distractions and more internal silence.

Dr. Epstein recommends meditating for 20 minutes to an hour each day. But if you can't spare that much time, even 10 minutes can help. What's most important is getting in the habit of doing it on a daily basis, he says.

TAI CHI

What It Is

Tai chi is an ancient Chinese martial art. But unlike its more aggressive cousin, karate, it does not involve any violent chops or flying kicks. Instead, this gentle discipline combines a series of fluid, dancelike movements with meditative attention to the breath and body.

In San Francisco, tai chi classes congregate in the rectangular oasis of landmark Golden Gate Park, which stretches from midtown to the seashore. Since they were immortalized in Armistead Maupin's book series (and TV miniseries) *Tales of the City*, the great flocks of tai chi enthusiasts have become something of a tourist attraction.

The graceful pattern of tai chi seems right at home in an outdoor setting. Preparing for class, the students stand with relaxed knees, as silent as the shadows moving over the grass. Beginning the individual movements traditionally called forms, they raise and lower their arms and legs in slow synchronicity, mimicking tree branches swaying in the breeze.

Even the names of the tai chi exercises echo nature: "grasp the bird's tail," "wind blows lotus leaves," "wave hands like clouds." The exercises themselves are poetically gentle, with knees bent and unlocked, wrists loose, and hands relaxed and open. Because the ending position of one form serves as the starting position for the subsequent form, tai chi is like a smooth, slow dance routine, only without the music.

What It Does

In China, tai chi has a longstanding reputation as a healing discipline. "It is real medicine," affirms Martin Inn, O.M.D., a doctor of oriental medicine and founder of and teacher at the Inner Research Institute of Tai Ji Quan in San Francisco. Tai chi is prescribed not only for arthritis but also for heart trouble, depression, and insomnia, to name just a few ailments.

In fact, the health benefits of tai chi rival those of high-intensity Western exercise. Tai chi, however, delivers its therapeutic punch via mechanisms that are the complete opposite of sweaty, heart-pounding aerobic workouts. "Standard aerobic exercise stresses the body, raising the heart rate, constricting blood vessels, and increasing tension," Dr. Inn notes. "Its effects are similar to those of the classic fight-or-flight response."

Tai chi puts a stop to the stress cycle, Dr. Inn explains. It quiets the body's emergency response system, allowing blood and oxygen to flow freely. And this tonic effect is only one of tai chi's benefits. Here are several more.

Relieves chronic joint pain. In a study involving 16 people with arthritis, those who attended weekly hour-long tai chi classes reported significantly less pain than those who didn't take the classes. Tai chi helps by increasing blood flow to the joints, which reduces inflammation and eases joint pain and stiffness. In addition, the range of motion required by tai chi exercises improves flexibility in the joints. This preserves mobility—and may help prevent arthritis in the first place.

Strengthens muscles. Regular tai chi practice is a gentle technique for building musculoskeletal strength. "The movements themselves are very slow," says Lixing Lao, Ph.D., assistant professor in the complementary medicine program at the University of Maryland School of Medicine in Baltimore and a tai chi instructor. "But slow exercise actually is more challenging to bones and muscles." And because tai chi works the arms, legs, and torso equally, it benefits muscle groups throughout the body.

Improves balance. An impaired sense of balance leads to a higher risk of falls. For older people, even one tumble could cause debilitating damage. Research has shown that tai chi may significantly reduce the likelihood of losing balance.

One particular study involving 200 people, all at least 70 years of age, compared tai chi with computerized balance training. After 15 weeks, those practicing tai chi were 47.5 percent less likely to experience frequent falls than those receiving computerized training.

Enhances mood. Tai chi is good for the mind as well as the body. Research has shown that it can lift the spirits, leaving tension, depression, and anger in the lurch. One study, conducted at the University of

Massachusetts Medical School in Worcester, found
that 16 weeks of tai chi beat the blues more effectively
than the same amount of walking. "Tai chi seems to
help uncover hidden emotions, releasing psychologi-
cal tension," notes Nikki Winston, a tai chi instructor
at the Golden Door Spa in Escondido, California, and
at Win International in Delmar, California.

Start Something!

You can learn tai chi by enrolling in a class—many
health clubs, YM/YWCAs, and churches offer them—
or by watching an instructional video. Even if you're
a veteran tai chi student, you may be able to get more
from your sessions by heeding this expert-
recommended advice.

Go with the flow. Think of tai chi as slow solo
dancing, a series of steps linked together to form a
cohesive, fluid routine. "Remember to keep moving
as you practice," Winston says. "If you stay in a particular pose, you may become tense. And that's not
what tai chi is about."

Have fun. An attitude of playfulness can help ban-
ish any self-consciousness about practicing tai chi. "In
China, people often say, 'Let's play tai chi,' " Winston notes. They perform their exercises with a combination of expressiveness and exuberance. You can
too, just by relaxing and enjoying yourself.

Set a standing appointment. To see results
quickly, your best bet is to plan for at least one tai
chi session a day, Dr. Lao says. If your schedule
doesn't allow it, then aim for at least two or three
sessions a week. Keep in mind that you don't need to

set aside a big block of time. Just 20 minutes per session should do the trick.

Tune in to your body. If you experience any pain while practicing tai chi, stop your exercises right away. Seek medical attention if the problem seems severe. "You should never experience even a moment of discomfort," Winston says. "Tai chi is about feeling better all over, not worse."

Trial Run

If you'd like to sample a tai chi–style exercise, get ready for the "tai chi cheer." Winston adapted this simple movement from traditional Asian forms. It can "open the body and the heart," she says, helping to counteract the closed state so often associated with pain and depression. Here's what to do.

- Stand in a relaxed position with your knees slightly bent.
- Holding your hands just below your belly button, place one on top of the other, with both palms facing upward.
- Take a normal step forward with your right foot, putting all of your weight on that foot. Rise onto the toes of your left foot.
- As your legs move, open your arms and hands downward toward the earth in an expansive gesture. Remain in this open position for one full inhalation and exhalation.
- Step back, returning your arms to the starting position.
- Step forward again, this time raising your arms

straight out to the sides. "Really open your
arms wide," Winston says. "Imagine that you
are opening your heart." Hold this position for
one full inhalation and exhalation.
- Step back, returning your arms to the starting
position.
- Step forward onto your right foot and open
your arms high overhead. As you reach for the
sky, let out a loud cheer, such as "Yay!" or even
"Aahhh!"
- Step back, then repeat the entire exercise, this
time leading with your left foot.

"Everyone loves the tai chi cheer," Winston says.
"You can't help but feel more lighthearted after doing
it."

YOGA

What It Is

Despite its name, this ancient Indian discipline has
absolutely nothing to do with former baseball great
Yogi Berra or cartoon great Yogi Bear. *Yoga*—the
word is Sanskrit for "to join"—blends deep breathing,
stretching, and meditation to bring into harmony a
person's physical, mental, and spiritual selves.

A typical yoga class lasts from an hour to an hour
and a half. Students wear loose, comfortable clothing,
minus socks and shoes. And they don't necessarily sit
in the infamous lotus position, with their legs en-
twined so that the tops of both feet rest high on the
opposite thighs. For beginners especially, sitting

Indian-style is much more comfortable—and more realistic.

Some teachers like to begin class with a round of breathing exercises called *pranayama*. These exercises help to clear the mind and the lungs. The class then moves to the physical poses, or asanas. While some—like the headstand or the full wheel (a complete back bend, with hands and feet on the floor)—are quite challenging, a good teacher will start with the basics. The class ends with a period of deep relaxation to calm the mind and, in theory, allow the body to reap the most benefit from the poses.

Usually, the relaxation component centers on *savasana*, or the corpse pose. In savasana, students lie on their backs with their arms resting alongside their bodies and their legs and feet about hip-width apart. With their eyes closed and their muscles unwound, their minds can focus and become completely still. Some teachers feel savasana is the most difficult of the yoga poses because it requires complete relaxation of every part of the body, which is easier said than done.

What It Does

At its most basic, yoga is tranquility training. It's so effective because it requires such sharp concentration and focus, says Lee Lipsenthal, M.D., vice president and medical director of the Preventive Medicine Research Institute in Sausalito, California.

If this seems contradictory, consider the soothing effect of having a hobby. "Whenever people focus intently on one thing—be it painting model airplanes, planting a garden, or something else—they tend to become calm," Dr. Lipsenthal observes. "Two or three hours can just fly by."

Taming tension is just one of yoga's multiple health-enhancing effects. Another is that it reduces levels of key stress hormones called catecholamines. Because catecholamines appear to impair the activity of white blood cells, the soldiers of the immune system, controlling the hormones through regular yoga practice may enhance immune function. That's good for virtually every system in the body, Dr. Lipsenthal says.

Besides preventing asthma attacks, relieving digestive complaints, and improving sexual performance, yoga has some very specific benefits for arthritic joints. For starters, the slow stretching involved in the yoga poses improves flexibility and range of motion. "You may manage only a tiny stretch the first time you try it," Dr. Lipsenthal says. "But keep at it, and you'll notice a profound difference in the long run."

What's more, yoga poses loosen up the muscles and tendons that support the joints. This separates the bones in the joints and keeps them from rubbing together—especially important for osteoarthritis, the wear-and-tear form of the disease.

Start Something!

Yoga's potential rewards are many. But as the saying goes, you've got to play to win. With these tips, you can get in the game.

Invest in lessons. If you're new to yoga, you ought to enroll in a class, if only to learn proper technique. Otherwise, you could risk an injury. Many health clubs and YM/YWCAs offer classes, as do churches and community colleges.

Even if you take a class, try to practice at home every day, advises Rodney Yee, director of the Piedmont Yoga Studio in Oakland, California, and producer of numerous yoga videotapes. A 10- to 15-minute session should be enough—though feel free to go longer, if you have time.

Stick with it. Unless you make a serious commitment to yoga, you may not realize any benefits from it. Give it 6 months, Yee suggests. "After 6 months of consistent practice, you'll be in a place where you really *want* to make time for it," he says. Indeed, you may wonder how you got by without it for so long!

Trial Run

So you say you've been out of commission because of your arthritis? Not exercising very much, if at all? Yoga may be the perfect discipline for easing back into an active lifestyle.

One particularly user-friendly variation is Easy Does It Yoga (EDY), developed by Alice Christensen, founder and executive director of the American Yoga Association in Sarasota, Florida. Intended for seniors and those with physical limitations, EDY has the same basic components as traditional yoga: breathing exercises, poses, and relaxation or meditation. The key difference is that the poses are done in bed or seated in a chair, at least to start. As a person's strength and balance improve, standing poses and floor work are added to the routine.

Easy Does It Yoga may be especially beneficial for those with arthritis, because it helps loosen stiff, achy joints, Dr. Lipsenthal says. To get a feel for the simple but effective EDY poses, try the seated leg lift.

- Take off your shoes and sit in a sturdy, armless chair with your lower back against the backrest and both feet flat on the floor. Grasp the sides of the seat with your hands.
- Take three slow, deep breaths, inhaling and exhaling fully. On the fourth inhalation, straighten your right knee and raise your leg as high as you can without straining. Push your heel away from your body while pulling your toes toward you.
- Hold for a count of three or as long as is comfortable, then exhale while lowering your leg. Relax and breathe normally.
- When you're ready, repeat the sequence with your left leg. Then continue alternating until you've completed three repetitions with each leg.

PART IV

Your Outsmart Arthritis Plan

CHAPTER TEN

7 Days to Healthier Joints

This Sunday, plan on going to the playground and swinging with your kids or grandkids, sitting down with them to a spaghetti dinner, and not having one moment of irritation or anger. That's what you'll do on the very first day of this weeklong program.

Sounds doable, doesn't it? Maybe even fun?

Believe it or not, those activities—combined with a special diet and exercise plan—can help reduce your risk of or speed your recovery from arthritis as well as heart disease, cancer, diabetes, and osteoporosis. That's right: One program fights five major health problems in just 1 week!

As a bonus, this program can help you take off any extra pounds. It's an important benefit because obesity—which affects one in four American adults—is a major risk factor for arthritis. It also can aggravate existing joint problems.

HOW IT WORKS

The following pages spell out all the details of the program. We start it on a Sunday, but you can pick any day. To help track your progress, we've included a simple checklist with each day, so you can mark down all that you've eaten and all that you've done to stay active and reduce stress.

Each day of the program consists of two basic components. The first offers a series of easy-to-follow tips targeting diet ("On Your Plate"), exercise ("Get Fit Fast"), and stress management ("On Your Mind"). You also get to sample an alternative remedy ("Try an Alternative"), entice your taste buds ("Indulge"), engage your sense of play ("Have Fun!"), and pamper your joints ("Especially for Arthritis"). Must you do all of these things? No. Our hope is that you'll try at least one thing every day.

The second component features a strength-building exercise and a stretch. Ideally, you'll pair these with an aerobic activity of your choice. Together, they'll improve your strength and flexibility—which is essential for healthy joints—and reduce your risk of injury. They'll also support weight loss, if that's your goal.

YOUR DIET PLAN

To complement the 7 days of lifestyle strategies in the following pages, we've put together a diet plan to cover your body's nutritional needs. You can use the checklist that accompanies each day to tally your food

servings, as well as your supplement doses. Here are
the basic guidelines.

1. Eat Nine Servings of Fruits and Vegetables Each Day

This may seem tough, but it really isn't. After all, a
typical serving consists of ½ cup of fruit or vegetable
or ¾ cup of juice. Have a banana—which counts as
2 servings—and a glass of OJ with your morning cereal, and you're one-third of the way to your daily
quota. (For a complete rundown of serving sizes, see
"How Much Is a Serving?" on page 118.)

Why nine a day and not five, as the popular slogan
recommends? The five-a-day campaign aims to convince people to eat just one more serving of fruit or
veggie than they usually do. But you have good reason not to settle for the bare minimum.

Fruits and vegetables are treasure troves of antioxidants, which can help prevent the cellular damage
caused by naturally occurring molecules called free
radicals. Numerous studies have linked diets rich in
fruits and veggies with a lower risk of osteoarthritis,
as well as heart disease, cancer, diabetes, and even
osteoporosis. The landmark DASH study (Dietary Ap-
proaches to Stop Hypertension) found that people who
ate an average of nine servings a day could lower their
blood pressure as effectively as with some prescription drugs.

HOW MUCH IS A SERVING?

The recommended number of servings for each food group may seem like a lot. But as you can see in this list, the actual serving sizes are rather small. So they add up quickly.

FRUITS AND VEGETABLES
- ½ cup chopped fruit
- 1 medium piece of whole fruit
- ½ cup cooked or raw vegetables
- 1 cup raw greens
- ¾ cup vegetable or fruit juice

WHOLE GRAINS
- 1 slice whole wheat bread
- ½ cup brown rice or bulgur
- ½ cup whole wheat pasta

HIGH-CALCIUM FOODS
- 1 cup fat-free or 1 percent milk
- 1 cup fat-free or low-fat yogurt
- 1 ounce reduced-fat cheese
- 1 cup calcium-fortified orange juice

BEANS
- ½ cup cooked dried beans or lentils

NUTS
- 2 tablespoons, chopped

FISH
- 3 ounces, cooked

2. Eat Three to Six Servings of Whole Grain Foods Each Day

People who eat an abundance of whole grains are less likely to experience heart disease, stroke, cancer, and diabetes than people who eat refined carbohydrates like breads, bagels, crackers, and rolls made with white flour. Unfortunately, refined carbs are staples in the standard American diet.

Your body recognizes refined carbohydrates as sugar, which raises your insulin levels—a known risk factor for heart disease and diabetes. And the latest research suggests that a diet rich in refined carbs can increase a woman's risk for breast cancer by 40 percent. On the other hand, a diet rich in whole grains and fiber can protect against colon and other cancers.

Don't rely on color to distinguish a whole grain from a refined one. Some brown breads, for example, actually use white flour. Instead, make sure the word *whole* precedes any grain mentioned in the ingredients list.

3. Eat Two or Three Servings of Calcium-Rich Foods Each Day

You already may be watching your calcium intake to protect your bones against osteoporosis. But did you know that calcium also helps prevent colon cancer, high blood pressure, and PMS? According to new research, drinking milk may reduce a woman's risk of breast cancer, too.

Choose fat-free and 1 percent milk, low-fat and fat-

free yogurt, and reduced-fat and fat-free cheeses over
the full-fat varieties. If you're lactose intolerant, look
for lactose-free dairy products, or get your calcium
from calcium-fortified juice or soy milk. To match the
amount of calcium in regular milk, a food should supply at least 30 percent of the Daily Value of calcium
per serving. Check the nutrition label.

4. Eat at Least Five Servings of Beans Each Week

Except for wheat bran, no food contains more fiber
than beans. Diets rich in fiber are associated with a
lower incidence of heart disease, stroke, cancer, and
diabetes. The soluble fiber found in beans is especially
good at helping to lower cholesterol.

Beans also are a good source of folate, a B vitamin
that reduces levels of homocysteine. Like high cholesterol, a high level of homocysteine is a risk factor
for heart disease.

Since beans come in cans, they're very easy to prepare. Just be sure to rinse off the canning liquid,
which contains a lot of sodium.

5. Eat Five Servings of Nuts Each Week

The monounsaturated fats in nuts are better for your
joints, not to mention your heart, than the polyunsat-
urated fats in corn and safflower oils. People who eat
nuts regularly are less likely to develop heart disease
and other illnesses than people who don't. But moderation is key, as nuts are high in calories. Keep a jar

of chopped nuts in your fridge, and sprinkle 2 table-spoons a day on vegetables, cereal, salad, or yogurt.

6. Eat Two Servings of Fish Each Week

Some research evidence suggests that fish may help treat some forms of arthritis, as well as depression and a digestive ailment called Crohn's disease. Fish also supplies omega-3 fatty acids, the beneficial fats known to lower the risk of heart attack deaths. The fish species with the most omega-3's include salmon, white albacore tuna, rainbow trout, anchovies, herring, sardines, and mackerel.

7. Drink 8 to 10 Glasses of Water, Plus 1 Cup of Tea, Each Day

Tea—both green and black—may help protect against rheumatoid arthritis, heart disease, and cancer. As for water, people who drink lots of it seem less likely to develop colon and bladder cancers.

8. Keep a Fat Budget

Many experts advise getting no more than 25 percent of your calories from fat. But just how much is that?

First, you need to calculate how many calories you can consume on a daily basis. For women who want to lose weight, the usual recommendation is between 1,500 and 1,800 calories a day, with a minimum of 1,200. Men who are slimming down typically need between 2,000 and 2,300 calories a day, with a minimum of 1,600. Which end of the calorie range you aim for depends on how active you are; the more exercise you do, the more calories your body burns.

Second, once you've determined your ideal calorie intake, you can use the following chart to determine your fat budget, in grams. You can find out the number of fat grams in various foods by reading the nutrition labels.

Calories	Fat Grams
1,250	35
1,500	42
1,750	49
2,000	56
2,300	64

You need some fat in your diet to help absorb fat-soluble nutrients. But try to get most of it from monounsaturated fats and omega-3 fatty acids such as olive and canola oils, nuts, and fish. If you use margarine, look for one that doesn't contain trans fats, which can raise cholesterol. Avoid products that have "partially hydrogenated" anything in their ingredients lists.

9. Take a Multivitamin Each Day

While you'll be getting a healthy mix of nutrients from your diet, you can cover your nutritional bases by taking a multivitamin-mineral supplement plus 100 to 500 milligrams of vitamin C and 100 to 400 IUs of vitamin E every day. On those days when you eat only two servings of calcium-rich foods, get an extra 500 milligrams of the mineral in supplement form.

10. Make Wise Choices

The beauty of this diet plan is that you can eat virtually anything you want—even the following "forbidden" foods. Again, moderation is key.

Meat and poultry: You can have up to 3 ounces—a serving roughly the size of a deck of cards—each day. Actually, if you stick with the rest of the dietary guidelines, you'll be getting plenty of protein. So you could cut back on your meat consumption. Studies have shown that vegetarians tend to be healthier, possibly because their no-meat diets are lower in saturated fat.

Eggs: If you are overweight or you have diabetes or high cholesterol, you should limit yourself to four eggs a week. Otherwise, you can eat up to seven a week.

Sweets: Sugary foods should be once-in-a-while treats, because they're loaded with empty calories. Try to satisfy your sweet tooth with fruit or low-fat, calcium-rich ice cream and yogurt.

Alcohol: While it's good for the heart, alcohol may slightly raise the risk of breast cancer. Limit yourself to one drink a day if you're a woman, two a day if you're a man. A drink equals 12 ounces of regular beer, 5 ounces of wine, or a cocktail made with 1½ ounces of 80-proof distilled spirits.

YOUR EXERCISE PLAN

Along with a sensible diet, regular exercise is vital for flexible, pain-free joints and overall good health. Being unfit can raise your risk for heart disease, cancer, diabetes, and even early death. Research has shown that very fit men are likely to live nearly 9 years longer than unfit men.

"Low cardiorespiratory fitness is as hazardous as cigarette smoking," according to Steven Blair, P.E.D. (physical education doctor), director of research at the Cooper Institute for Aerobics Research in Dallas. In some cases, being fit actually can counteract the health risks associated with smoking, being overweight, or having high cholesterol, blood pressure, or blood sugar levels.

If you've been relatively sedentary, walking may be the best activity for easing into your exercise plan. You don't need any special equipment other than a good pair of walking shoes. And you can do it practically anywhere. Aim for just 10 minutes a day to start. Then slowly work up to 30 to 60 minutes of moderate-intensity activity—such as walking, jogging, stair-climbing, cycling, or swimming—at least 5 days a week. You may want to extend your workouts if you're trying to lose weight.

In addition to aerobic exercise, we recommend 20 to 30 minutes of strength training 2 or 3 days a week. To make this more manageable, we've included a strength-training session in each day of the program. If you're new to strength training, do just the "For Starters" exercise. As you get stronger, or if you're looking for faster results, you can add on the "More Challenging" exercise. And don't forget the stretch!

Be sure to check with your doctor before you begin exercising, especially if you've been inactive or you have a physical problem that could complicate your fitness routine. And take time to ease into it, to protect your joints and reduce your risk of injury.

DAY ONE: SUNDAY

On Your Plate

Bring on the marinara. Men who eat more tomato sauce are less likely to develop prostate cancer, probably because of a pigment in tomatoes called lycopene. Think more sauce, less spaghetti.

Get Fit Fast

Do two. Can't fit an entire strength-training routine into your schedule? Do just two exercises every day, so by week's end, you will have hit all your major muscle groups. It takes less than 10 minutes, yet it keeps those muscles—and bones—strong.

On Your Mind

Stamp out hissy fits! Getting steamed can double your risk of having a heart attack within the subsequent 2 hours. Vow that just for today, no matter what goes wrong, you won't get angry. Instead, ask yourself these questions:

- Is what's upsetting me really important?
- Is what I'm thinking and feeling appropriate to what happened?
- Can anything I do change the situation?
- Is what I want to do worth the cost?

SUNDAY'S CHECKLIST

Mark each box as you fulfill each recommendation. Fill in the blanks where appropriate.

DAILY SERVINGS
- ☐ 5 vegetables
- ☐ 4 fruits
- ☐ 3–6 whole grains
- ☐ 2 or 3 high-calcium foods
- ☐ 8–10 glasses of water
- ☐ 1 cup of tea

WEEKLY SERVINGS
- ☐ 5-plus beans
How many? _____
- ☐ 5 nuts
How many? _____
- ☐ 2 fish
How many? _____

SUPPLEMENTS
- ☐ Multivitamin/mineral containing 100 percent of the Daily Values for most nutrients
- ☐ Vitamin C: 100–500 mg
- ☐ Vitamin E: 100–400 IU
- ☐ Calcium: 500 mg

EXERCISE
- ☐ Aerobic (30 minutes)
What activity? _____
- ☐ Strength training
- ☐ Stretching
- ☐ Relaxation
What activity? _____

Try an Alternative

Add garlic to your shopping list. The next time you hit the natural foods supermarket, pick up a tub of freshly peeled garlic cloves and challenge yourself to use all of it before the "best by" date. The payoff? A healthy heart and possibly a reduced risk of cancer.

Indulge

Try a papaya. This sweet tropical fruit is rich in soluble fiber, which can help lower your blood sugar.

Have Fun!

Go swinging. A half-hour of pumping your legs to fly high on a swing burns more than 100 calories and works both the front and back of your thighs. If you push someone else, your biceps get a good workout, too.

Especially for Arthritis

Stay seated. If you're experiencing an arthritis flare-up, or if you have severe hip or knee damage or balance problems, try exercising while sitting in a chair. It's better than not exercising at all.

Today's Exercise

For starters: The Side Lunge strengthens and tones your quadriceps and inner thighs. Do one set of 10 repetitions, counting 1-2-3 as you lunge and 1-2-3 as you return to the starting position.

Stand with your feet as far apart as possible and your hands on your hips. Turn your right foot to the side, then twist your upper body in the direction of your right foot. Bend your right knee until you can see only the tips of your right toes. Your left leg should stay extended. Pause, then return to the starting position. Complete one set, then switch legs.

More challenging: For total leg toning, try the Single Leg Squat. It targets the quads as well as the glutes (the muscles in the hips and buttocks) and hamstrings. It also improves balance. Do one set of 10 repetitions, counting 1-2-3 as you lower and 1-2-3 as you return to the starting position.

Stand with your feet slightly apart, lightly resting your hands on the back of a chair for support. Raise your left leg behind you about 30 to 45 degrees. Bend your right leg, lowering your body a few inches. Make sure you can see your toes below your knee. Pause before returning to the starting position. Complete a set, then switch legs.

Stretch it out: Flexible muscles feel better and appear longer, hence leaner. This stretch relaxes the muscles running down the back of your legs.

Place your hands on the back of a chair. Slowly walk your legs back until your body forms a right angle. Press your heels into the ground, and lift your buttocks toward the ceiling. Hold for 10 to 30 seconds.

DAY TWO: MONDAY

On Your Plate

Make time for your morning meal. Even if you're dieting, don't skip breakfast. A survey of more than 2,000 people who lost an average of 67 pounds and kept off the weight for more than 5 years found that 78 percent eat breakfast every day of the week. Only 4 percent skip it entirely.

Get Fit Fast

Put down that paper! If you pare 2 minutes from reading the newspaper, you'll free up time for two sets of crunches. Shave 5 minutes from scanning e-mails or paging through the *TV Guide*, and you can squeeze in a workout on a stair-climbing machine. Watch for those inactive minutes in your daily routine and use them to do something—*anything*. Eventually, you'll be in motion for an extra 10, 15, even 20 minutes each day.

On Your Mind

Ask the Big Questions. Find a time and a place to sit undisturbed. Then grab a pen and paper, and jot down your thoughts on the following questions: Why are you here? What gifts do you give to the world? What does God want you to do in this life? The answers may not come easy, but they can reveal what's meaningful in your life. They also counteract negative

MONDAY'S CHECKLIST

Mark each box as you fulfill each recommendation. Fill in the
blanks where appropriate.

DAILY SERVINGS
☐ 5 vegetables
☐ 4 fruits
☐ 3–6 whole grains
☐ 2 or 3 high-calcium foods
☐ 8–10 glasses of water
☐ 1 cup of tea

WEEKLY SERVINGS
☐ 5-plus beans
How many? _____
☐ 5 nuts
How many? _____
☐ 2 fish
How many? _____

SUPPLEMENTS
☐ Multivitamin/mineral containing 100 percent of the Daily
   Values for most nutrients
☐ Vitamin C: 100–500 mg
☐ Vitamin E: 100–400 IU
☐ Calcium: 500 mg

EXERCISE
☐ Aerobic (30 minutes)
What activity? _____
☐ Strength training
☐ Stretching
☐ Relaxation
What activity? _____

feelings that may be suppressing your immune function.

Try an Alternative

Tug yourself out of bed. It's Monday morning, and you just don't want to get out from under the covers. So grab yourself by the ears. By gently tugging around the tops and pulling along the lobes, you'll stimulate acupuncture points that provide more energy to start your day.

Indulge

Take the Subway. Jared, the guy who lost so much weight eating Subway sandwiches, is on to something. A 6-inch Subway Veggie has only 200 calories and 2.5 grams of fat. Yet it supplies 3 grams of fiber and 40 percent of the Daily Value of vitamin C. So why not go out to lunch today?

Have Fun!

Do a quick burn. Want to use up 100 calories without setting foot on a treadmill? You can do it with 29 minutes of miniature golf, 22 minutes of fly-fishing, or 18 minutes of gardening.

Especially for Arthritis

Treat yourself to satin pj's. Rolling over in bed will be slippery-smooth, reducing nightly discomfort and ensuring a solid night's sleep. If you can't find satin pajamas at a local department store, take your search online. Many online catalogs carry them.

Today's Exercise

For starters: The Lateral Raise is a simple shoulder-builder that makes your arms look great. Do one set of 10 repetitions, counting 1-2-3 as you lift and 1-2-3 as you lower. Use weights heavy enough to make the last few reps feel tough.

Stand with your feet shoulder-width apart, dumbbells at your sides. Keeping your elbows slightly bent, raise the dumbbells outward until your arms are parallel to the floor. Pause before returning to the starting position.

More challenging: Get super shoulder strength with the Lying Rear Fly. Do one set of 10 repetitions, counting 1-2-3 as you lift and 1-2-3 as you lower. Use weights heavy enough to make the last few reps feel tough.

Lie facedown with your chin resting lightly on the floor. Holding a dumbbell in each hand, extend your arms out to the sides, keeping your palms down and your elbows slightly bent. Squeeze your shoulder blades together as you slowly raise your arms a few inches. Pause before returning to the starting position.

Stretch it out: Everyday tasks are easier with supple shoulders. This stretch helps keep your deltoid muscles relaxed. Standing with your feet apart, extend both arms in front of you. Use your right hand to gently guide your left elbow across your body. Keep your shoulders and shoulder blades down. Hold for 15 to 60 seconds, then switch arms and repeat.

TUESDAY'S CHECKLIST

Mark each box as you fulfill each recommendation. Fill in the blanks where appropriate.

DAILY SERVINGS
- [ ] 5 vegetables
- [ ] 4 fruits
- [ ] 3–6 whole grains
- [ ] 2 or 3 high-calcium foods
- [ ] 8–10 glasses of water
- [ ] 1 cup of tea

WEEKLY SERVINGS
- [ ] 5-plus beans

How many? _____
- [ ] 5 nuts

How many? _____
- [ ] 2 fish

How many? _____

SUPPLEMENTS
- [ ] Multivitamin/mineral containing 100 percent of the Daily Values for most nutrients
- [ ] Vitamin C: 100–500 mg
- [ ] Vitamin E: 100–400 IU
- [ ] Calcium: 500 mg

EXERCISE
- [ ] Aerobic (30 minutes)

What activity? _____
- [ ] Strength training
- [ ] Stretching
- [ ] Relaxation

What activity? _____

DAY THREE: TUESDAY

On Your Plate

Have an Italian dessert. Visit Italy, and you'll see mostly slim people. One big reason: For dessert, they have fruit. Tonight, instead of three chocolate chip cookies, eat a peach. Make a similar trade every day for a year, and you'll lose more than 12 pounds.

Get Fit Fast

Declare this no-TV Tuesday. One day a week, keep the TV and computer turned off. Fill that time by doing something active—perhaps playing with the kids or grandkids, or just dancing around your living room. Once you see how good you feel, it may become a habit you look forward to.

On Your Mind

Be different. Do something you've never done before, just for yourself. See one of the Harry Potter movies. Paint your toenails orange. Get up and sing in a karaoke bar. It not only fights depression, it also stimulates your mind—which in turn stimulates immune function.

Try an Alternative

Mix and match herbal immune-boosters. An array of herbs—including astragalus, maitake, and echinacea—stoke your immune system. Choose one to take three times each day, or switch between several.

Indulge

Snack on shrimp. Twelve large shrimp contain only 65 calories.

Have Fun!

Stay well-connected. Join a group that walks, runs, bikes, uses pogo sticks—whatever. You'll get support and motivation to stay active, plus all the health benefits associated with being around other people.

Especially for Arthritis

Heat things up. No more "It hurts too much to walk in the morning" excuses! Invest in an electric blanket or mattress pad, and turn it on before you get out of bed. It's guaranteed to melt away that morning stiffness.

Today's Exercise

For starters: Strong glutes make jeans look good and climbing stairs a snap. Start toning with the Leg Pulse. Do one set of 10 repetitions, counting 1-2-3 as you lift and 1-2-3 as you lower.

Standing with your feet together, raise your left leg straight behind you until it's several inches off the floor. (If you're concerned about losing your balance, be sure you're near a wall to catch yourself.) Tighten your butt muscles, and press your left leg back even farther. Pause before returning to the starting position. Complete a set, then switch legs.

More challenging: Give your glutes extra lift with the Kick Back. Do one set of 10 repetitions, counting 1-2-3 as you lift and 1-2-3 as you lower.

Begin on your hands and knees, with your head in line with your spine. Contract your glutes, and move your left leg backward until your thigh is parallel to the floor. Your left knee should remain bent. Pause before returning to the starting position. Complete a set, then switch legs.

Stretch it out: Tight glutes can contribute to lower back discomfort. This stretch helps prevent tightening. Holding on to a door frame or railing, cross your left foot over your right knee so that your left knee points out to the left. Sit back until your right thigh is almost parallel to the floor. Hold for 15 to 60 seconds, then switch legs.

DAY FOUR: WEDNESDAY

On Your Plate

Wrap it up! As mentioned earlier, beans are loaded with fiber and the B vitamin folate, which helps prevent heart attacks and fight birth defects. It also may protect against Alzheimer's disease. For a fast and tasty dinner for two, mix a 16-ounce can of black beans and a 16-ounce can of corn (both drained) with 1 to 2 cups of spicy tomato salsa. Divide between 2 or 3 whole wheat tortillas, wrap, and enjoy.

WEDNESDAY'S CHECKLIST

Mark each box as you fulfill each recommendation. Fill in the blanks where appropriate.

DAILY SERVINGS
- [ ] 5 vegetables
- [ ] 4 fruits
- [ ] 3–6 whole grains
- [ ] 2 or 3 high-calcium foods
- [ ] 8–10 glasses of water
- [ ] 1 cup of tea

WEEKLY SERVINGS
- [ ] 5-plus beans

How many? _____
- [ ] 5 nuts

How many? _____
- [ ] 2 fish

How many? _____

SUPPLEMENTS
- [ ] Multivitamin/mineral containing 100 percent of the Daily Values for most nutrients
- [ ] Vitamin C: 100–500 mg
- [ ] Vitamin E: 100–400 IU
- [ ] Calcium: 500 mg

EXERCISE
- [ ] Aerobic (30 minutes)

What activity? _____
- [ ] Strength training
- [ ] Stretching
- [ ] Relaxation

What activity? _____

Get Fit Fast

Practice the rule of 10. Don't feel like exercising today? Set your watch alarm or a timer for 10 minutes at the start of your workout. If you want to quit after 10 minutes, go ahead. Chances are, you'll feel so good that you'll keep moving.

On Your Mind

String some beads. Studies have shown that prayer can reduce the risk of high blood pressure and heart attack. So why not make your own prayer beads? Buy beads and string at your local craft store, then slide one bead on the string for each person or issue you want to pray for or just think about. If you're not a particularly religious person, simply sit quietly for 10 minutes twice each day.

Try an Alternative

Chase away that midafternoon slump. Add a few drops of peppermint essential oil to a mister filled with cool water. When fatigue sets in, shake the bottle, shut your eyes, and spritz!

Indulge

Don't be afraid of the dark. If you have a hankering for chocolate, choose the dark variety. It contains more antioxidants than Concord grape juice.

Have Fun!

Drag out the old two-wheeler. Riding a bicycle helps shape your butt and tone your legs. As a bonus, you can burn about 475 calories in an hour.

Especially for Arthritis

Soothe achy joints gingerly. A teaspoon of grated fresh ginger in a cup of boiling water makes a refreshing tea that may help relieve arthritis pain. Fill a Thermos in the morning, and sip away all day.

Today's Exercise

For starters: The Modified Push-Up targets the chest muscles, or pectorals. While strong pecs may seem like a guy thing, they also benefit women by giving lift to the breasts. Do one set of 10 repetitions, counting 1-2-3 as you lower and 1-2-3 as you return to the starting position.

Begin on your hands and knees, with your head in line with your spine. Extend your right leg, and point your toes. Bend your elbows to lower your torso until your forehead is just above the floor. Pause before returning to the starting position. Switch legs, and repeat. If this move feels too difficult, keep both legs on the floor.

More challenging: Add curves to your chest with the Crisscross Fly. Do one set of 10 repetitions, counting 1-2-3 as you lift and 1-2-3 as you lower.

Lie on the floor or a bench with your knees bent and your feet flat on the floor. Holding dumbbells, extend your arms out to the sides, with your palms facing your feet. Raise the weights over your chest, crossing your arms at your elbows. Keep your elbows straight but not locked. Pause before returning to the starting position.

Stretch it out: Tight chest muscles can lead to slouching. The following stretch will help open up your chest.

Stand with your feet apart. Hold a towel behind your back, grasping it at the ends. Pull the towel taut, and gently lift up a little. (A longer towel makes the stretch easier.) Hold for 15 to 60 seconds.

DAY FIVE: THURSDAY

On Your Plate

Make the 25-pound switcheroo. Prevent heart attacks, strokes, cancer, and diabetes with one simple strategic change: Instead of a 20-ounce regular soda, drink water, sparkling water, unsweetened iced tea, or even diet soda or iced tea. You'll save 240 calories a day. Do it for a year, and you'll drop 25 pounds!

Get Fit Fast

Get in gear with gear. A heart rate monitor can make sure you're exercising intensely enough to get results, without overdoing it. A pedometer might provide the necessary inspiration to squeeze more steps into your day. Giant exercise balls can work your

THURSDAY'S CHECKLIST

Mark each box as you fulfill each recommendation. Fill in the blanks where appropriate.

DAILY SERVINGS
- [ ] 5 vegetables
- [ ] 4 fruits
- [ ] 3–6 whole grains
- [ ] 2 or 3 high-calcium foods
- [ ] 8–10 glasses of water
- [ ] 1 cup of tea

WEEKLY SERVINGS
- [ ] 5-plus beans

How many? _____

- [ ] 5 nuts

How many? _____

- [ ] 2 fish

How many? _____

SUPPLEMENTS
- [ ] Multivitamin/mineral containing 100 percent of the Daily Values for most nutrients
- [ ] Vitamin C: 100–500 mg
- [ ] Vitamin E: 100–400 IU
- [ ] Calcium: 500 mg

EXERCISE
- [ ] Aerobic (30 minutes)

What activity? _____

- [ ] Strength training
- [ ] Stretching
- [ ] Relaxation

What activity? _____

muscles in myriad ways. Request a catalog from the Walker's Warehouse (an affiliate of *Prevention* magazine) by calling (888) 972–9255 or logging on to www.walkerswarehouse.com.

On Your Mind

Be thankful. Gratitude is a stress reliever. Make a list of all your blessings. As you open your eyes this morning, take a deep breath and say "I am." Then as you exhale, say "grateful."

Try an Alternative

Hang out at the water cooler. Taking your immune-boosting herbs? Well, you'd better be drinking your eight glasses of water, too. Herbal remedies work best when your body is well hydrated.

Indulge

Make a sticky snack. Fill 4 large pitted dates with 2 tablespoons of peanut butter. Studies have shown that people who regularly eat peanut butter are more likely to stick with their diets and less likely to develop heart disease.

Have Fun!

Go shoe shopping. Buy an extra pair of walking shoes to keep in your office or your car, so you can rack up some mileage whenever you get a chance.

Especially for Arthritis

Make it a joint venture. Contact the Arthritis Foundation for its brochure *51 Ways to Be Good to Your Joints*, filled with tips for maintaining healthy joints. Call (800) 283–7800, or visit www.arthritis.org.

Today's Exercise

For starters: Almost everyone has back pain at some point in their lives. But you can beat the odds, and improve your posture, by strengthening your back muscles. The Plank is the perfect exercise for doing this. It targets your lower back muscles, as well as your abs and glutes.

Lie facedown on the floor, with your legs extended and your feet flexed. Rise onto your forearms so that your elbows are directly beneath your shoulders. Then lift your body to form a straight line from your shoulders to your feet. Hold for 15 seconds before returning to the starting position. Repeat four times.

More challenging: For a more advanced move to strengthen your lower back muscles, try the Chest Lift. Do one set of 10 repetitions, counting 1-2-3 as you lift and 1-2-3 as you lower.

Lie facedown on the floor with your hands under your chin. Lift your head, chest, and arms about 5 to 6 inches off the floor. Pause before returning to the starting position.

Stretch it out: To avoid injury and stay pain-free, your back needs to be flexible as well as strong. This stretch is an ideal complement to any back exercise. Begin on your hands and knees. Pull in your abs, then round your back toward the ceiling while dropping your head toward the floor. Hold for 15 to 60 seconds.

DAY SIX: FRIDAY

On Your Plate

Go grain hunting. Eating whole grains lowers your risk of colon cancer in part because they contain powerful antioxidants, which may help prevent other forms of cancer as well. As pointed out earlier, you need to read ingredients lists to be sure you're getting whole grains. With breads, you may be able to see the grains in the loaves.

Get Fit Fast

Hit the weights. If you must choose between aerobic exercise and strength training—because you have limited time, for example—go with strength training. You likely will see faster results with just two sessions a week, which can help maintain your motivation. One study found that strength training could improve cardiovascular fitness as much as walking. And as you get stronger, everyday tasks will be easier. So naturally, you'll be more active.

On Your Mind

Visualize a healthy heart. Zap the effects of stress on your heart with some guided imagery from thera-

FRIDAY'S CHECKLIST

Mark each box as you fulfill each recommendation. Fill in the blanks where appropriate.

DAILY SERVINGS
- ☐ 5 vegetables
- ☐ 4 fruits
- ☐ 3–6 whole grains
- ☐ 2 or 3 high-calcium foods
- ☐ 8–10 glasses of water
- ☐ I cup of tea

WEEKLY SERVINGS
- ☐ 5-plus beans
How many? _____
- ☐ 5 nuts
How many? _____
- ☐ 2 fish
How many? _____

SUPPLEMENTS
- ☐ Multivitamin/mineral containing 100 percent of the Daily Values for most nutrients
- ☐ Vitamin C: 100–500 mg
- ☐ Vitamin E: 100–400 IU
- ☐ Calcium: 500 mg

EXERCISE
- ☐ Aerobic (30 minutes)
What activity? _____
- ☐ Strength training
- ☐ Stretching
- ☐ Relaxation
What activity? _____

pist Belleruth Naparstek. Play her 50-minute CD or audiotape *Healthy Heart*, and feel your heart open to better health. To order, call (800) 800-8661, or visit www.healthjourneys.com.

Try an Alternative

Get a garlic gadget. Make health-promoting garlic an easy addition to any meal with a great kitchen tool. The Zyliss Garlic Press removes the peel and crushes the garlic in one easy motion. To find a store near you, call (888) 794–7623, or visit the company Web site at www.zylissusa.com.

Indulge

Use your noodles. Serve up some comfort food tonight with a single-serving side dish of Stouffer's Macaroni and Cheese Dinner, tossed with 1 pound of cooked broccoli florets. It makes 4 servings of about 1⅓ cup, each with 244 calories, 12 grams of fat, 5 grams of saturated fat, and 4 grams of fiber. You can have it for lunch, too.

Have Fun!

Hear a pin drop. Instead of seeing a movie tonight, go bowling. It burns three times more calories than sitting in a theater. And if you're bad at it, it's funnier than a Jim Carrey flick.

Especially for Arthritis

Join a mall-walking club. Walking is an ideal exercise for most people, including most arthritis sufferers. If you have severe hip, knee, ankle, or foot problems, talk with your doctor before you start. For tips on getting fit at the mall, check out *Mall Walking Madness* by Sara Donovan. It's available wherever books are sold, by calling (800) 848–4735, or by logging on to www.rodalestore.com.

Today's Exercise

For starters: The Triceps Kickback is a simple solution for strong, jiggle-proof arms. Do one set of 10 repetitions, counting 1-2-3 as you lift and 1-2-3 as you lower. Use weights heavy enough to make the last few reps feel tough.

Bend over a chair seat, supporting yourself with your right hand. Your back should be flat. Grasp a dumbbell with your left hand, and place your left elbow at your side with your forearm perpendicular to the floor. Keeping your upper arm still, move your forearm backward until it is parallel to the floor. Pause before returning to the starting position.

More challenging: The Curl and Press targets the triceps, biceps, and shoulders. Do one set of 10 repetitions, counting 1-2-3-4-5 as you lift and 1-2-3-4-5 as you lower.

Sit in a chair, with your feet flat on the floor. Hold dumbbells at your sides, with your palms facing forward. Bend your elbows, and lift the weights toward your shoulders. Rotate your wrists so that your palms face forward, and raise the weights overhead. Pause, then work backward through the movements to the starting position.

Stretch it out: Flexible arms function better. This stretch helps keep your arms limber.

Raise your right arm overhead. Bend your right elbow, and reach down the middle of your back with your right hand. Your right elbow should point toward the ceiling. With your left hand, gently press your right elbow into a deeper but not uncomfortable stretch. Hold for 15 to 60 seconds, then switch arms.

DAY SEVEN: SATURDAY

On Your Plate

Bag it. Going out for dinner? Restaurant portions can be enormous. Counting every course, from appetizer through dessert, you should eat no more than 2½ cups of food. For a visual comparison, that's a little more than a pint carton of milk. Once you reach that amount, request a doggie bag for the rest.

Get Fit Fast

Step outside. A stimulating environment serves as a distraction, so you work harder without realizing it. In one study, gardening burned nearly 30 percent more calories than indoor aerobics: 392 calories versus 306. Other research has shown that walkers subconsciously pick up their pace outdoors.

SATURDAY'S CHECKLIST

Mark each box as you fulfill each recommendation. Fill in the blanks where appropriate.

DAILY SERVINGS
- ☐ 5 vegetables
- ☐ 4 fruits
- ☐ 3–6 whole grains
- ☐ 2 or 3 high-calcium foods
- ☐ 8–10 glasses of water
- ☐ 1 cup of tea

WEEKLY SERVINGS
- ☐ 5-plus beans
How many? _____
- ☐ 5 nuts
How many? _____
- ☐ 2 fish
How many? _____

SUPPLEMENTS
- ☐ Multivitamin/mineral containing 100 percent of the Daily Values for most nutrients
- ☐ Vitamin C: 100–500 mg
- ☐ Vitamin E: 100–400 IU
- ☐ Calcium: 500 mg

EXERCISE
- ☐ Aerobic (30 minutes)
What activity? _____
- ☐ Strength training
- ☐ Stretching
- ☐ Relaxation
What activity? _____

On Your Mind

Forgive their trespasses. If you feel bitter toward someone who has wronged you, you're just letting that person hurt you again: The resulting stress hormones can increase your risk of a heart attack fivefold. Make an effort to let bygones be bygones.

Try an Alternative

Put magnets on the soles of your shoes. In a small but well-controlled study, people with diabetic neuropathy found pain relief from magnetic insoles. In the study, participants used Magsteps insoles by Nikken. To order, call (888) 264–5536, or visit the company's Web site at www.nikken.com.

Indulge

Order the lobster. Sweet Maine lobster has only 83 calories per 3-ounce serving—even less than skinless turkey breast. Just skip the melted butter!

Have Fun!

Think about sex. Studies have shown that just thinking about sex or romance can reduce pain and improve mood. What happens after that is up to you.

Especially for Arthritis

Upgrade your kitchen. These days, you can outfit your kitchen with a variety of products that enhance accessibility and support mobility for arthritic joints. Look for rollout baskets, step-up shelf extenders, wire dividers, and easy-to-grip kitchen utensils. For more ideas, visit The Container Store at www.thecontainer store.com, Bed Bath & Beyond at www.bedbathand beyond.com, or Organized Living at www.organized living.com.

Today's Exercise

For starters: The Standing Twist is an easy way to firm a soft midsection without getting on the floor. Do one set of 10 repetitions on each side, counting 1-2-3 as you lift and twist and 1-2-3 as you return to the starting position.

Stand with your feet a few inches apart. Bend your arms, and hold them out to the sides, at right angles to your body. Your hands should point toward the ceiling, with your palms facing forward. Contract your abs, and pull your right knee and left elbow toward one another. Pause before returning to the starting position. Complete a set, then switch sides.

More challenging: For more advanced toning, try the Crunch and Reach to target all of the abdominal muscles. Do one set of 10 repetitions on each side, counting 1-2-3 as you lift and 1-2-3 as you lower.

Lie on your back, with your arms extended overhead and your legs extended at almost 90 degrees to your body. Tighten your abs, and lift your head and shoulders off the floor, pressing your hands toward your feet. Pause, then lower.

Stretch it out: Like other muscles, abs need a good stretch after strength training. This one should do the trick. Lie facedown with your feet together and your toes pointed. Your palms should be on the floor, just in front of your shoulders. Lift your chin, and gently raise your head and chest off the floor as far as comfortable. Hold for 15 to 60 seconds.

CHAPTER ELEVEN

Recipes That Heal

This chapter features a collection of tasty recipes brimming with irresistible flavors—not to mention key nutrients that may help fight arthritis. Many of these dishes supply healthy doses of vitamin C and other antioxidants, which neutralize cell-damaging free radicals. Some are fantastic sources of omega-3 fatty acids, beneficial fats that effectively reduce inflammation. Some contain an abundance of fiber, which can help take off any extra pounds that may be taxing your joints.

For good measure, we've made all of these recipes low in saturated fat, a harmful fat that can trigger arthritis flare-ups. Saturated fat also contributes to heart disease and diabetes, among other ailments. So by incorporating these dishes into your diet, you'll be doing your whole body a world of good. Enjoy!

BREAKFASTS

The most important meal of the day, breakfast jump-starts your energy and stabilizes your blood sugar, which helps prevent overeating—a major factor in weight gain—later in the day. Of course, these recipes are chock-full of nutrients that your joints will love!

Orange-Bran Muffins

The Healing Factor: Excellent source of omega-3 fatty acids, vitamin C, and fiber

2 cups shredded all-bran cereal

¾ cup hot water

¼ cup canola oil

1 orange

¾ cup buttermilk

2 tablespoons light molasses

2 tablespoons honey

1 egg

1¼ cups whole grain pastry flour

⅓ cup + 2 teaspoons rolled oats

2 teaspoons baking soda

½ teaspoon salt

1 cup raisins

¼ cup chopped toasted walnuts (optional)

¼ cup sugar

¼ cup orange juice

Preheat the oven to 400°F. Coat a 12-cup muffin pan with cooking spray.

In a medium bowl, combine the cereal, water, and oil. Stir until the cereal is softened.

Grate 1 tablespoon of the peel from the orange into another medium bowl; cut the orange in half and squeeze ¼ cup of juice into the bowl. Stir in the buttermilk, molasses, honey, and egg until well-blended. Stir into the cereal mixture.

In a large bowl, combine the flour, ⅓ cup of the oats, baking soda, and salt. Add the cereal mixture and stir just until blended. Stir in the raisins and walnuts, if using.

Divide the batter evenly among the prepared muffin cups. Sprinkle with the remaining 2 teaspoons oats. Bake for 15 minutes, or until a wooden pick inserted in the center of a muffin comes out clean. Place the pan on a rack to cool.

Meanwhile, combine the sugar and orange juice in a small saucepan. Bring to a boil over medium heat and stir until the sugar dissolves. Using a wooden pick, poke holes in the muffin tops. Brush with the hot orange syrup.

Let the muffins cool on the rack for 5 minutes. Then remove them from the pan and place them directly on the rack to finish cooling.

Makes 12 muffins
Per muffin: 220 calories, 5 g protein, 42 g carbohydrates, 6 g total fat, 1 g saturated fat, 18 mg cholesterol, 6 g fiber, 353 mg sodium

Honeyed Summer Fruit Bowl

The Healing Factor: Excellent source of vitamin C and a good source of fiber

¼ cup honey

1 tablespoon lemon juice or lime juice

Pinch of ground cinnamon

1½ pints strawberries, quartered

½ large cantaloupe, cut into chunks or balls

2 medium nectarines, cut into thin wedges

   2 medium peaches, cut into thin wedges
   2 large or 3 small plums, cut into thin wedges
   1 cup blueberries

In a large bowl, combine the honey, lemon juice or lime juice, and cinnamon. Add the strawberries, cantaloupe, nectarines, peaches, plums, and blueberries. Toss just until the fruit is well-mixed and coated with the honey mixture.

   Let stand for 30 minutes before serving to allow the flavors to blend.

Makes 8 servings

Per serving: 112 calories, 1 g protein, 28 g carbohydrates, 1 g total fat, 0 g saturated fat, 0 mg cholesterol, 3 g fiber, 5 mg sodium

Fiesta Cornmeal Pudding

The Healing Factor: Excellent source of vitamin C and a good source of fiber

   2¼ cups water
   ½ teaspoon salt
   ¾ cup yellow cornmeal
   1 tablespoon extra-virgin olive oil
   1 large red bell pepper, chopped
   4 scallions, thinly sliced
   2 large cloves garlic, minced
   1 package (10 ounces) frozen chopped spinach, thawed and squeezed dry
   2 egg whites
   ¼ teaspoon hot-pepper sauce
   ½ cup (2 ounces) shredded sharp Cheddar cheese

Preheat oven to 350°F. Coat a 9-inch baking dish with cooking spray.

Bring the water to a boil in a large saucepan over high heat. Add the salt. Reduce the heat to medium-low. Add the cornmeal in a slow, steady stream, whisking constantly. Reduce the heat to low, cover, and cook, stirring frequently, for 10 minutes, or until very thick. Remove from the heat.

Meanwhile, heat the oil in a medium nonstick skillet over medium heat. Add the bell pepper; cook, stirring, for 4 minutes. Add the scallions and garlic; cook, stirring, for 2 minutes, or until the vegetables are tender. Add the bell pepper mixture, spinach, egg whites, and hot-pepper sauce to the cornmeal. Stir well. Place in the baking dish. Sprinkle with the cheese. Bake for 30 minutes, or until firm, puffed, and golden.

Makes 6 servings

Per serving: 145 calories, 7 g protein, 17 g carbohydrates, 6 g total fat, 2 g saturated fat, 10 mg cholesterol, 3 g fiber, 323 mg sodium

Florentine Omelette

The Healing Factor: Excellent source of vitamin C

2 eggs

2 egg whites

3 tablespoons water

1 teaspoon dried Italian seasoning, crushed

1/4 teaspoon salt

8 ounces mushrooms, sliced

1 onion, chopped

1 red bell pepper, chopped

1 clove garlic, minced

4 ounces (2 packed cups) spinach leaves, chopped

3/4 cup (3 ounces) shredded low-fat mozzarella cheese

Preheat the oven to 200°F. Coat a baking sheet with cooking spray.

In a medium bowl, whisk together the eggs, egg whites, water, Italian seasoning, and salt.

Coat a large nonstick skillet with cooking spray and place over medium-high heat. Add the mushrooms, onion, pepper, and garlic and cook, stirring often, for 4 minutes, or until the pepper starts to soften. Add the spinach and cook for 1 minute, or until the spinach is wilted. Place in a small bowl and cover.

Wipe the skillet with a paper towel. Coat with cooking spray and place over medium heat. Pour in half of the egg mixture. Cook for 2 minutes, or until the bottom begins to set. Using a spatula, lift the edges to allow the uncooked mixture to flow to the bottom of the pan. Cook for 2 minutes longer, or until set. Sprinkle with half of the reserved vegetable mixture and half of the cheese. Cover and cook for 2 minutes, or until the cheese melts. Using a spatula, fold the egg mixture in half. Place on the prepared baking sheet and place in the oven to keep warm.

Coat the skillet with cooking spray. Repeat with the remaining egg mixture, vegetable mixture, and cheese to cook another omelette. To serve, cut each omelette in half.

Makes 4 servings

Per serving: 128 calories, 13 g protein, 7 g carbohydrates, 7 g total fat, 3 g saturated fat, 115 mg cholesterol, 3 g fiber, 346 mg sodium

SALADS

Salads are a lunch mainstay because they're so fast and easy. But they make an excellent meal at any time of day. Be creative with the ingredients, sampling the variety of greens and the exotic fruits and vegetables now available in most supermarkets. Experimenting adds excitement to healthy eating—so you're more likely to stick with it!

Strawberry and Red Onion Salad

The Healing Factor: Excellent source of vitamin C and fiber and a good source of omega-3 fatty acids

3 tablespoons strawberry all-fruit spread

2 teaspoons balsamic vinegar

1 teaspoon olive oil

1 teaspoon flaxseed oil

1/8 teaspoon salt

1/8 teaspoon crushed red-pepper flakes

1 pound fresh strawberries, hulled and sliced

1/4 cantaloupe, cut into 1/4-inch chunks

1/2 small red bell pepper, finely chopped

1/2 small red onion, finely chopped

1 medium head escarole, torn (about 3 cups)

1/2 ripe avocado, cut into 1/4-inch chunks

Freshly ground black pepper

In a medium glass bowl, combine the all-fruit spread, vinegar, olive oil, flaxseed oil, salt, and red-pepper flakes until well-blended. Gently fold in the strawberries, cantaloupe, bell pepper, and onion. Cover and let stand for 15 minutes to allow the flavors to blend.

Place the escarole in a serving bowl. Add the avocado and strawberry mixture and toss to coat well. Season with black pepper to taste.

Makes 4 servings

Per serving: 163 calories, 2 g protein, 27 g carbohydrates, 7 g total fat, 1 g saturated fat, 0 mg cholesterol, 6 g fiber, 110 mg sodium

Mediterranean Chickpea Salad

The Healing Factor: Excellent source of vitamin C and a good source of fiber

1 can (15 ounces) chickpeas, rinsed and drained

3 plum tomatoes, chopped

2 roasted red peppers, chopped

1/2 small red onion, quartered and thinly sliced

1/2 cucumber, peeled, halved, seeded, and chopped

2 tablespoons chopped parsley

2 cloves garlic, chopped

3 tablespoons lemon juice

1 1/2 teaspoons extra-virgin olive oil

1 1/2 teaspoons flaxseed oil

1/4 teaspoon salt

In a large bowl, combine all the ingredients. Toss to coat well. Let stand for at least 15 minutes to allow the flavors to blend.

Makes 8 servings

Per serving: 104 calories, 4 g protein, 18 g carbohydrates, 3 g total fat, 0 g saturated fat, 0 mg cholesterol, 4 g fiber, 158 mg sodium

Balsamic Tomato and Roasted Pepper Salad

The Healing Factor: Excellent source of vitamin C

1 1/2 teaspoons balsamic vinegar

1 teaspoon extra-virgin olive oil

1 teaspoon flaxseed oil

1 small clove garlic, minced

1/4 teaspoon salt

1/8 teaspoon freshly ground black pepper

2 large red bell peppers, halved and seeded

2 large tomatoes, cut into 1/2-inch thick slices
1/3 cup julienne-cut fresh basil leaves

Preheat the broiler. Coat a broiler-pan rack with cooking spray.

In a cup, whisk together the vinegar, olive oil, flaxseed oil, garlic, salt, and pepper; set aside.

Place the bell peppers, skin side up, on the prepared rack. Broil, without turning, for 8 to 12 minutes, or until the skins are blackened and blistered in spots.

Place the peppers in a bowl and cover with a kitchen towel. Let stand for 10 minutes, or until cool enough to handle. Peel the skin from the peppers and discard. Cut the peppers into 1/2-inch wide strips.

Arrange the tomato slices on a platter. Scatter the pepper strips on top and sprinkle with the basil. Drizzle the dressing over the salad. Let stand for at least 15 minutes to allow the flavors to blend.

Makes 4 servings

Per serving: 53 calories, 1 g protein, 8 g carbohydrates, 3 g total fat, 0 g saturated fat, 0 mg cholesterol, 2 g fiber, 153 mg sodium

SOUPS

By blending a variety of vegetables—often with meat, poultry, or fish—hot and hearty soup can deliver an entire meal's worth of nutrients in one satisfying bowl. Feel free to substitute your favorite veggies for those listed in the recipes. While we've recommended specific amounts for many of the herbs and spices, you're welcome to use more, if you wish. After all, these seasonings add flavor without fat or sodium. As a bonus, many of them are chock-full of healing phytonutrients.

Curried Sweet Potato and Apple Soup

The Healing Factor: Excellent source of vitamin C and good source of fiber

I tablespoon olive oil
I large onion, sliced
2 cloves garlic, sliced
I tablespoon finely chopped fresh ginger
I teaspoon curry powder
¾ teaspoon ground cumin
½ teaspoon salt
¼ teaspoon ground cinnamon
4 cups water
I ¼ pounds sweet potatoes, peeled and cut into chunks
3 large Granny Smith apples, peeled, cored, and cut into chunks
½ cup chopped fresh cilantro

Heat the oil in a large saucepan or Dutch oven over medium heat. Add the onion and garlic and cook, stirring occasionally, for 5 minutes, or until tender.

Add the ginger, curry powder, cumin, salt, and cinnamon. Cook, stirring constantly, for I minute. Add the water, sweet potatoes, and apples and bring to a boil over high heat. Reduce the heat to low, cover, and simmer, stirring often, for 20 minutes, or until the sweet potatoes are very tender.

In a food processor or blender, puree the soup in batches until very smooth, pouring each batch into a bowl. Reheat if necessary. Stir in the cilantro.

Makes 8 servings
Per serving: 134 calories, 2 g protein, 29 g carbohydrates, 2 g total fat, 0 g saturated fat, 0 mg cholesterol, 4 g fiber, 162 mg sodium

Minestrone Verde

The Healing Factor: Excellent source of vitamin C and a good source of fiber

2 teaspoons extra-virgin olive oil

2 small leeks, white and green parts, halved lengthwise, rinsed, and thinly sliced

2 large ribs celery with leaves, thinly sliced

2 cloves garlic, minced + 1 whole clove garlic, peeled

1/4 teaspoon dried oregano, crushed

1/4 teaspoon freshly ground black pepper

1/8 teaspoon salt

2 cups water

1 cup chicken broth

4 cups chopped Swiss chard

1/8 cup frozen baby lima beans

1/4 cup ditalini or other small pasta

1/4 cup chopped Italian parsley

1/2 cup frozen green peas

4 teaspoons shredded Parmesan cheese (see note)

Heat the oil in a large saucepan over medium heat. Add the leeks, celery, minced garlic, oregano, pepper, and salt. Cook, stirring frequently, for 4 minutes, or until the vegetables begin to soften.

Add the water, broth, Swiss chard, lima beans, and pasta. Bring to a boil over high heat. Reduce the heat to medium-low, cover, and simmer for 8 minutes, or until the vegetables are tender and the pasta is al dente.

Meanwhile, coarsely chop the remaining garlic clove, then mince it together with the parsley. Stir the garlic-parsley mixture and the peas into the soup. Cover and cook for 5 minutes, or until the peas are heated through.

Ladle the soup into 4 bowls and top each with 1 teaspoon of the cheese.

Makes 4 servings

Per serving: 145 calories, 6 g protein, 24 g carbohydrates, 3 g total fat, 1 g saturated fat, 1 mg cholesterol, 5 g fiber, 413 mg sodium

Health note: People with depression who take monoamine oxidase inhibitors (MAO inhibitors) should avoid alcohol and other fermented or aged products, such as the cheese in this recipe.

Seven-Bean Soup with Greens

The Healing Factor: Excellent source of vitamin C and fiber

⅓ cup black beans
⅓ cup red kidney beans
⅓ cup appaloosa or small red beans
⅓ cup cranberry or pinto beans
⅓ cup great Northern or navy beans
⅓ cup Steuben yellow-eye beans or black-eyed peas
3 tablespoons extra-virgin olive oil
10 cloves garlic, minced
2 large onions, coarsely chopped
2 ribs celery, sliced
2 teaspoons dried Italian herb seasoning, crushed
¾ teaspoon freshly ground black pepper
⅓ cup green or yellow split peas
6 cups water
2 cans (28 ounces each) crushed tomatoes in tomato puree

¼ cup tomato paste
2 packages (10 ounces each) frozen chopped greens, such as collard, turnip, or kale
½ teaspoon salt
1½ cups chopped fresh basil

Pick over and rinse all the beans. Place in a large saucepot and cover with 3 inches of water. Cover and let stand overnight. Drain.

Rinse and dry the pot. Heat the oil in the pot over medium-high heat. Add the garlic, onions, and celery and cook, stirring frequently, for 5 minutes, or until soft. Add the Italian seasoning and pepper and cook, stirring, for 30 seconds.

Add the beans, split peas, and water. Bring to a boil over high heat. Reduce the heat to medium-low, cover, and simmer, stirring occasionally, for 1½ hours, or until the beans are tender. (The black beans will take the longest to cook, so use them as a guide.)

Add the tomatoes, tomato paste, greens, and salt. Bring to a boil over high heat. Reduce the heat to medium-low, cover, and simmer, stirring occasionally, for 30 minutes longer, or until the greens are tender. Stir in the basil.

Makes 8 servings
Per serving: 349 calories, 19 g protein, 56 g carbohydrates, 6 g total fat, 1 g saturated fat, 0 mg cholesterol, 18 g fiber, 688 mg sodium

Split Pea Soup with Ham and Winter Squash
The Healing Factor: Excellent source of vitamin C and fiber
1 smoked ham hock (12 ounces)
11 cups water
4 cloves garlic, minced

 1 teaspoon dried thyme, crushed
 1/2 teaspoon dried sage, crushed
 1/2 teaspoon freshly ground black pepper
 1 pound green split peas, picked over and rinsed
 1 medium butternut squash (2 pounds), peeled and cut into 1/2-inch chunks
 1 pound white potatoes, scrubbed and cut into 1/2-inch chunks
 3 large carrots, cut into 1/2-inch chunks
 3 ribs celery, sliced
 2 large onions, coarsely chopped
 3/4 teaspoon salt

In a large saucepot or Dutch oven, combine the ham hock, water, garlic, thyme, sage, and pepper. Bring to a boil over high heat. Reduce the heat to low, cover, and simmer, turning the ham hock once, for 1 hour. Cool. Refrigerate for at least 4 hours or overnight.

After the broth has chilled, skim and discard the fat from the surface. Remove the ham hock and cut the meat off the bone; set aside. Discard the bone and any fat.

Add the split peas to the broth and bring to a boil over high heat. Skim off any foam that rises to the surface. Reduce the heat to low, cover, and simmer, stirring occasionally, for 1 hour, or until the peas are soft and tender.

Add the squash, potatoes, carrots, celery, onions, salt, and ham. Return to a boil. Cover and simmer, stirring occasionally, for 20 to 25 minutes, or until the vegetables are tender.

Makes 8 servings
Per serving: 350 calories, 20 g protein, 64 g carbohydrates, 3 g total fat, 1 g saturated fat, 7 mg cholesterol, 19 g fiber, 464 mg sodium

Root Vegetable Soup

The Healing Factor: Excellent source of vitamin C and fiber

1 tablespoon olive oil

6 cloves garlic, minced

2 large onions, chopped

1/2 teaspoon dried marjoram, crushed

1/2 teaspoon dried sage, crushed

1/4 teaspoon salt

1/2 teaspoon freshly ground black pepper

1 pound lean, well-trimmed beef round, cut into 1-inch cubes

3 cups low-sodium beef broth

3 cups water

1 can (28 ounces) whole tomatoes, drained and broken up

4 small turnips, peeled and cut into 1/2-inch chunks

3 medium beets, peeled and cut into 1/2-inch chunks

3 large carrots, cut into 1/2-inch chunks

2 medium parsnips, peeled and cut into 1/2-inch chunks

Heat the oil in a large saucepan over medium heat. Add the garlic and onions and cook, stirring, for 5 minutes, or until soft. Add the marjoram, sage, salt, and pepper. Add the beef and cook, stirring, for 5 minutes, or until browned.

Add the broth, water, and tomatoes. Bring to a boil over high heat. Reduce the heat to low, cover, and simmer, stirring occasionally, for 45 minutes, or until the beef is very tender.

Add the turnips, beets, carrots, and parsnips. Return to a simmer. Cover and cook, stirring occasionally, for 25 minutes longer, or until the vegetables are very tender.

Makes 6 servings
Per serving: 311 calories, 24 g protein, 36 g carbohydrates, 7
g total fat, 2 g saturated fat, 36 mg cholesterol, 9 g fiber, 583
mg sodium

GRAINS AND LEGUMES

Grains and legumes are nutritional powerhouses.
They're packed with complex carbohydrates, fiber, vitamins, and minerals, yet they contain very little fat
and sodium and no cholesterol. These days, whole
grains—the healthiest kind—are widely available.
Even better, they're inexpensive and easy to use. Experiment with grains ranging from the familiar brown
rice to the out-of-the-ordinary quinoa. As for legumes,
they come in all shapes and sizes, tastes and textures.
Fill your shelves with a large selection of canned and
dried varieties.

Cilantro and Tomato Rice
The Healing Factor: Excellent source of vitamin C and fiber

1 cup short-grain rice
2 cups water
1/2 teaspoon salt
1 pound tomatoes, coarsely chopped
1/3 cup chopped fresh cilantro
1 tablespoon extra-virgin olive oil
1 tablespoon lime juice or lemon juice
1 clove garlic, minced
1 teaspoon ground cumin
1/4 teaspoon freshly ground black pepper
1 can (14–19 ounces) chickpeas, rinsed and drained
1/4 cup slivered almonds, toasted

Place the rice, water, and ¼ teaspoon of the salt in a medium saucepan. Bring to a boil over high heat. Reduce the heat to low, cover, and simmer for 50 minutes, or until the rice is tender and the liquid is absorbed.

Meanwhile, in a medium bowl, combine the tomatoes, cilantro, oil, lime juice or lemon juice, garlic, cumin, pepper, and the remaining ¼ teaspoon salt. Cover and let stand at room temperature. Stir in the rice and chickpeas and top with the almonds.

Makes 4 servings

Per serving: 405 calories, 12 g protein, 68 g carbohydrates, 11 g total fat, 1 g saturated fat, 0 mg cholesterol, 10 g fiber, 472 mg sodium

Polenta with Fresh Tomato Sauce

The Healing Factor: Excellent source of vitamin C and fiber

6 cups water

¾ teaspoon salt

2 cups coarse yellow cornmeal

½ cup (2 ounces) freshly grated Parmesan cheese (see note)

1 tablespoon extra-virgin olive oil

1 large clove garlic, minced

¼ teaspoon dried oregano, crushed

¼ teaspoon fennel seeds, crushed

8 plum tomatoes, coarsely chopped

⅛ teaspoon freshly ground black pepper

2 tablespoons tomato paste

Preheat the oven to 400°F. Coat a 9- by 9-inch baking dish with cooking spray. Bring the water to a boil in a large saucepan over high heat. Stir in ½ teaspoon of the salt. Add the cornmeal in a slow, steady stream, whisking constantly. Bring to a boil. Stir in the cheese.

Remove from the heat and pour into the prepared baking dish. Bake for 35 minutes, or until firm.

Meanwhile, heat the oil in a large nonstick skillet over medium heat. Add the garlic, oregano, and fennel seeds and cook, stirring, for 3 minutes, or until fragrant.

Stir in the tomatoes, remaining ¼ teaspoon salt, and pepper. Increase the heat to high and bring to a boil. Reduce the heat to medium-low and simmer, stirring frequently, for 8 minutes, or until the tomatoes are cooked down and juicy. Add the tomato paste and cook, stirring, for 2 minutes, or until the sauce is slightly thickened. Cover and keep warm.

Serve the polenta with the sauce.

Makes 6 servings

Per serving: 246 calories, 8 g protein, 40 g carbohydrates, 7 g total fat, 2 g saturated fat, 7 mg cholesterol, 5 g fiber, 497 mg sodium

Health note: People with depression who take monoamine oxidase inhibitors (MAO inhibitors) should avoid alcohol and other fermented or aged products, such as the cheese in this recipe.

Garlic and Red Pepper Grits

The Healing Factor: Excellent source of vitamin C and omega-3 fatty acids and a good source of fiber

3 ¾ cups water

½ teaspoon salt

¾ cup quick-cooking grits

1 tablespoon canola oil

3 cloves garlic, minced

2 large red bell peppers, chopped

½ teaspoon paprika

½ teaspoon dried thyme, crushed

¼ teaspoon freshly ground black pepper
⅓ cup (1½ ounces) shredded Monterey Jack cheese

Bring the water to a boil in a medium saucepan over high heat. Add the salt and slowly stir in the grits. Reduce the heat to medium-low and cook, stirring occasionally, for 20 minutes, or until the grits are creamy and thickened. Remove from the heat.

Meanwhile, heat the oil in a medium nonstick skillet over medium-low heat. Add the garlic and cook, stirring, for 2 minutes, or until fragrant. Add the bell peppers, paprika, thyme, and black pepper and cook, stirring frequently, for 8 minutes, or until very tender. (Add a tablespoon of water to the pan if it gets dry.)

Stir the bell pepper mixture and cheese into the grits, stirring until the cheese melts.

Makes 4 servings
Per serving: 185 calories, 6 g protein, 27 g carbohydrates, 7 g total fat, 2 g saturated fat, 10 mg cholesterol, 3 g fiber, 358 mg sodium

Barley with Spring Greens
The Healing Factor: Excellent source of vitamin C and fiber
1½ cups chicken or vegetable broth
½ cup pearl barley
1 tablespoon extra-virgin olive oil
1 bunch scallions, thinly sliced
3 cloves garlic, slivered
10 cups loosely packed torn mixed greens, such as escarole, Swiss chard, watercress, and arugula
¼ teaspoon salt
⅛ teaspoon freshly ground black pepper

Bring the broth to a boil in a medium saucepan over high heat. Add the barley and return to a boil. Reduce the heat to low, cover, and simmer for 45 minutes, or until tender.

Meanwhile, heat the oil in a large saucepot or Dutch oven over medium-high heat. Add the scallions and garlic and cook, stirring frequently, for 3 minutes, or until the scallions are wilted.

Add the greens, salt, and pepper. Cook, stirring, for 3 minutes, or until just wilted.

Fluff the barley with a fork and stir into the greens.

Makes 4 servings
Per serving: 143 calories, 5 g protein, 24 g carbohydrates, 4 g total fat, 1 g saturated fat, 0 mg cholesterol, 7 g fiber, 391 mg sodium

VEGETABLES

From artichokes to squash, vegetables are a must for the nutrition-conscious. Like grains and legumes, veggies are rich in complex carbohydrates, fiber, vitamins, and minerals. As a bonus, they're very easy to prepare, and they're so versatile that you can enjoy a different vegetable-based dish every night of the week. While fresh veggies contain lots of nutrients, don't overlook frozen ones. Because they're picked and packaged at the peak of their season, frozen veggies pack plenty of nutritional muscle. They're great in the winter months, when fresh produce isn't as readily available.

Sweet Potato Stew
The Healing Factor: Excellent source of vitamin C and fiber
1½ cups uncooked brown rice

1 tablespoon olive oil

3 cloves garlic, minced

2 red bell peppers, cut into 1-inch chunks

1 large onion, chopped

1 tablespoon minced fresh ginger

1/2 teaspoon ground allspice

1/4 teaspoon ground red pepper

4 cups vegetable broth

2 large sweet potatoes, peeled and cut into 1-inch chunks

1/2 cup natural peanut butter

1 cup boiling water

1/3 cup tomato paste

1 can (10 1/2–15 ounces) chickpeas, rinsed and drained

1 pound spinach, coarsely chopped

Prepare the rice according to package directions.

Meanwhile, heat the oil in a Dutch oven over medium-high heat. Add the garlic, bell peppers, and onion; cook for 3 minutes. Add the ginger, allspice, and ground red pepper; cook for 1 minute.

Add the broth and potatoes; bring to a boil. Reduce the heat to low, cover, and simmer for 15 minutes, or until tender.

In a bowl, whisk the peanut butter and water. Add to the pan with the tomato paste, chickpeas, and spinach. Cook for 10 minutes, or until heated through. Serve over the rice.

Makes 6 servings

Per serving: 426 calories, 19 g protein, 61 g carbohydrates, 16 g total fat, 3 g saturated fat, 0 mg cholesterol, 16 g fiber, 669 mg sodium

Spicy Oven Fries

Healing Factor: Excellent source of vitamin C and omega-3 fatty acids

2 medium russet potatoes, scrubbed and cut into long, ½-inch thick strips

1 tablespoon canola oil

1 tablespoon roasted garlic and red pepper spice blend

¼ teaspoon salt

¼ teaspoon freshly ground black pepper

Preheat the oven to 425°F. Coat a 13- by 9-inch baking pan with cooking spray.

Place the potatoes in a mound in the prepared baking pan and sprinkle with the oil, spice blend, salt, and pepper. Toss to coat well. Spread the potatoes in a single layer.

Bake, turning the potatoes several times, for 40 minutes, or until crisp and lightly brown.

Makes 4 servings

Per serving: 115 calories, 3 g protein, 18 g carbohydrates, 4 g total fat, 0 g saturated fat, 0 mg cholesterol, 2 g fiber, 144 mg sodium

Stir-fried Asparagus with Ginger, Sesame, and Soy

The Healing Factor: Excellent source of vitamin C and omega-3 fatty acids

1½ pounds thin asparagus, cut diagonally into 2-inch pieces

2 teaspoons canola oil

½ large red bell pepper, cut into thin strips

1 tablespoon chopped fresh ginger

1 tablespoon reduced-sodium soy sauce (see note)

⅛ teaspoon crushed red-pepper flakes

1 teaspoon toasted sesame oil
1 teaspoon sesame seeds, toasted

Bring ¼ inch of water to a boil in a large nonstick skillet over high heat. Add the asparagus and return to a boil. Reduce the heat to low, cover, and simmer for 5 minutes, or until tender-crisp. Drain in a colander and cool briefly under cold running water. Wipe the skillet dry with a paper towel.

Heat the canola oil in the same skillet over high heat. Add the bell pepper and cook, stirring constantly, for 3 minutes, or until tender-crisp. Add the asparagus, ginger, soy sauce, and red-pepper flakes and cook for 2 minutes, or until heated through. Remove from the heat and stir in the sesame oil and sesame seeds.

Makes 4 servings

Per serving: 79 calories, 5 g protein, 7 g carbohydrates, 5 g total fat, 0 g saturated fat, 0 mg cholesterol, 4 g fiber, 157 mg sodium

Health note: People with depression who take monoamine oxidase inhibitors (MAOs) should avoid alcohol and other fermented or aged products, such as the soy sauce in this recipe. Substitute broth for the soy sauce.

Cinnamon Carrot Coins

The Healing Factor: Excellent source of vitamin C and a good source of fiber

6 medium carrots, thinly sliced
6 tablespoons orange juice
1½ teaspoons unsalted butter
¾ teaspoon ground cinnamon
⅛ teaspoon freshly ground black pepper

Place the carrots and orange juice in a medium saucepan. Cover and cook over medium-low heat for 6 minutes, or until the carrots are tender-crisp.

Add the butter, cinnamon, and pepper. Cook for 1 minute, stirring to coat.

Makes 4 servings

Per serving: 64 calories, 1 g protein, 12 g carbohydrates, 2 g total fat, 1 g saturated fat, 4 mg cholesterol, 3 g fiber, 33 mg sodium

Maple Squash with Cardamom

The Healing Factor: Excellent source of vitamin C and fiber

1 tablespoon butter, melted

1 tablespoon maple syrup

1 teaspoon ground cardamom

1/4 teaspoon salt

1 large butternut squash (3 1/4 pounds)

Preheat the oven to 400°F. Coat a 13- by 9-inch baking pan with cooking spray. In a large bowl, combine the butter, maple syrup, cardamom, and salt.

Pierce the squash in several places with a fork. Place in the microwave and cook for 4 minutes, or until softened. Peel and seed the squash and cut into 1-inch chunks. Add to the bowl with the butter mixture and toss to coat well. Place the squash mixture in the prepared baking pan.

Bake, tossing occasionally, for 45 minutes, or until browned and tender.

Makes 4 servings

Per serving: 207 calories, 4 g protein, 47 g carbohydrates, 3 g total fat, 2 g saturated fat, 8 mg cholesterol, 6 g fiber, 192 mg sodium

Vegetable Lasagna

The Healing Factor: Good source of vitamin C

1 teaspoon olive oil

1 zucchini, chopped

2 cups (16 ounces) reduced-fat ricotta cheese

1 egg

1 tablespoon dried basil

1/4 teaspoon salt

1 tablespoon ground black pepper

1 jar (16 ounces) spaghetti sauce

8 ounces no-cook lasagna (about 9 sheets)

10 ounces frozen broccoli, thawed

1 can (28 ounces) chopped tomatoes

1/4 cup (1 ounce) grated Parmesan cheese (see note)

1/4 cup (1 ounce) shredded reduced-fat mozzarella cheese

Preheat the oven to 350°F. Coat a 13- by 9-inch baking dish with nonstick spray.

Warm the oil in a medium skillet over medium heat. Add the zucchini and cook for 5 minutes, or until crisp-tender. Remove from the heat and set aside.

In a medium bowl, mix the ricotta, egg, basil, salt, and pepper. Set aside 1/2 cup of the spaghetti sauce.

Place 3 sheets of the lasagna in the prepared baking dish. Evenly spoon half of the remaining spaghetti sauce over lasagna. Top with half of the ricotta mixture, half of the broccoli, half of the zucchini, half of the tomatoes (with juice), and half of the Parmesan. Repeat layering with 3 more sheets of the lasagna and the remaining ingredients. End with the remaining sheets of lasagna. Spoon the reserved sauce over the top and sprinkle with the mozzarella.

Cover with foil and bake for 25 minutes. Uncover and

bake for 20 minutes, or until hot and bubbly. Let stand for 10 minutes before serving.

Makes 8 servings

Per serving: 212 calories, 15 g protein, 24 g carbohydrates, 6 g total fat, 43 mg cholesterol, 881 mg sodium, 4 g fiber

Health note: People with depression who take monoamine oxidase inhibitors (MAO inhibitors) should avoid alcohol and other fermented or aged products, such as the cheese in this recipe.

POULTRY AND FISH

Protein plays a vital role in building and repairing the body's tissues, which means it may help heal arthritic joints. Among protein sources, poultry and fish are healthier choices than red meat, because they tend to be lower in fat. But they're every bit as versatile, as the following recipes demonstrate.

Oven-Fried Chicken with Red Pepper-Sweet Onion Relish

The Healing Factor: Excellent source of vitamin C

Chicken

⅔ cup buttermilk or fat-free plain yogurt

2 tablespoons lime juice

½ teaspoon salt

½ teaspoon freshly ground black pepper

1¼ cups yellow cornmeal

1 cut-up chicken (3 pounds), wings saved for another use, skin and visible fat removed

Relish

1 large red bell pepper, finely chopped

1 small red onion, finely chopped

1/2 cup chopped fresh cilantro

2 tablespoons lime juice

1 tablespoon extra-virgin olive oil

1/8 teaspoon salt

To make the chicken: Preheat the oven to 425°F. Coat a large baking sheet with sides with cooking spray.

In a large bowl, combine the buttermilk or yogurt, lime juice, salt, and pepper. Place the cornmeal in a pie plate.

Dip the chicken in the buttermilk mixture, turning to coat well. (The chicken may be marinated in the buttermilk mixture in the refrigerator for up to 1 day.)

One at a time, roll the chicken pieces in the cornmeal, pressing to coat thoroughly. Place the chicken, skinned side up, on the prepared baking sheet. Discard any remaining buttermilk mixture and cornmeal.

Coat the chicken well with cooking spray. Bake for 40 minutes, or until a thermometer inserted in the thickest portion registers 170°F and the juices run clear.

To make the relish: Meanwhile, in a medium bowl, combine the bell pepper, onion, cilantro, lime juice, oil, and salt. Cover and let stand at room temperature.

Serve the chicken with the relish.

Makes 6 servings

Per serving: 399 calories, 52 g protein, 25 g carbohydrates, 9 g total fat, 2 g saturated fat, 161 mg cholesterol, 43 g fiber, 337 mg sodium

Chicken Piccata with Escarole

The Healing Factor: Excellent source of vitamin C

4 boneless, skinless chicken breast halves

½ teaspoon dried thyme, crushed

¼ teaspoon freshly ground black pepper

¼ teaspoon salt

2 cloves garlic, minced

5 cups loosely packed cut-up escarole

1 cup cherry tomatoes, halved

½ cup fat-free chicken broth

2 teaspoons cornstarch

½ teaspoon grated lemon peel

1 tablespoon lemon juice

1 tablespoon butter

Coat the broiler-pan rack with cooking spray. Preheat the broiler.

Season both sides of the chicken breasts with the thyme, pepper, and ⅛ teaspoon of the salt. Place the chicken on the broiler-pan rack and broil 2 to 3 inches from the heat for 5 minutes per side, or until a thermometer inserted in the thickest portion registers 160°F and the juices run clear. Place the chicken on a platter and keep warm.

Meanwhile, heat a large skillet coated with cooking spray over medium-high heat. Add the garlic and cook, stirring constantly, for 30 seconds, or until fragrant. Add the escarole and cook, stirring frequently, for 3 minutes, or until the greens begin to wilt. Add the tomatoes and the remaining teaspoon salt and cook for 3 minutes, or until the tomatoes are soft and the escarole is completely wilted. Place the vegetables on the platter with the chicken.

In a cup, combine the broth and cornstarch and stir until dissolved. In the same skillet, whisk together the cornstarch mixture, lemon peel, and lemon juice and bring to a boil over high heat, stirring constantly. Cook, stirring, for 1 minute, or until the sauce is slightly thickened. Add the butter and any juices that have collected on the platter and return to a boil, stirring constantly. Cook just until the butter is melted and the sauce has thickened. Pour the sauce over the chicken and vegetables.

Makes 4 servings
Per serving: 151 calories, 21 g protein, 6 g carbohydrates, 4 g total fat, 2 g saturated fat, 58 mg cholesterol, 3 g fiber, 257 mg sodium

---

Turkey and Bean Soft Tacos
The Healing Factor: Excellent source of vitamin C and fiber

8 corn tortillas (6-inch diameter)
8 ounces (2 cups) shredded cooked turkey breast
1 cup drained and rinsed canned kidney or pinto beans
1¼ cups mild or medium-spicy salsa + additional for topping
½ teaspoon ground cumin
1½ cups finely shredded cabbage
1 large carrot, shredded
¼ cup finely chopped sweet white onion
¼ cup reduced-fat cucumber ranch dressing

Preheat the oven to 350°F.

Stack the tortillas and wrap them in foil. Place the tortillas in the oven and heat for 10 minutes.

Meanwhile, heat a large skillet coated with cooking spray over high heat. Add the turkey, beans, 1¼ cups salsa, and cumin and bring to a boil. Reduce the heat to low, cover, and simmer, stirring for 10 minutes, or until heated through.

In a medium bowl, combine the cabbage, carrot, onion, and ranch dressing.

Spoon about ⅓ cup of the turkey filling into a tortilla. Top with ¼ cup of the cabbage mixture and fold over.

Repeat with the remaining tortillas, turkey filling, and cabbage mixture. Top each with the remaining salsa.

Makes 4 servings

Per serving: 330 calories, 24 g protein, 44 g carbohydrates, 6 g total fat, 1 g saturated fat, 47 mg cholesterol, 8 g fiber, 676 mg sodium

Pesto Salmon

The Healing Factor: Excellent source of omega-3 fatty acids

1¼ cups loosely packed fresh basil

1 clove garlic

3 tablespoons chicken broth

1 tablespoon blanched slivered almonds

1 tablespoon lemon juice

2 teaspoons freshly grated Parmesan cheese (see note)

2 teaspoons extra-virgin olive oil

¼ teaspoon salt

¼ teaspoon freshly ground black pepper

1 pound skinned salmon fillet, cut into 4 pieces

Lemon wedges (optional)

Basil sprigs (optional)

Place the fresh basil, garlic, broth, almonds, lemon juice, cheese, oil, salt, and pepper in a blender. Process until pureed.

Place the salmon on a plate. Spoon 3 tablespoons of the pesto over the salmon and turn to coat both sides. Cover with plastic wrap and let stand for 15 minutes. Reserve the remaining pesto.

Meanwhile, preheat the broiler. Spray a jelly-roll pan with cooking spray.

Place the salmon in the prepared pan. Spread any of the pesto remaining on the plate on top of each piece. Broil the salmon 4 to 5 inches from the heat for 6 to 8 minutes, or just until opaque.

Place the salmon pieces on 4 plates and top each piece with some of the reserved pesto. Garnish with lemon wedges and basil sprigs, if using.

Makes 4 servings

Per serving: 203 calories, 24 g protein, 2 g carbohydrates, 11 g total fat, 2 g saturated fat, 63 mg cholesterol, 1 g fiber, 242 mg sodium

Health note: People with depression who take monoamine oxidase inhibitors (MAO inhibitors) should avoid alcohol and other fermented or aged products, such as the cheese in this recipe.

Pan-Seared Red Snapper with Olive Crust

The Healing Factor: Excellent source of omega-3 fatty acids

1 cups fresh bread crumbs

1/4 cup chopped fresh oregano, basil, or thyme

16 pitted and finely chopped kalamata olives

2 tablespoons freshly grated Parmesan cheese (see note)

1/2 teaspoon freshly ground black pepper

4 red snapper fillets (5 ounces each)

In a shallow bowl, combine the bread crumbs; oregano, basil, or thyme; olives; cheese; and pepper. Firmly press the fillets into the mixture to coat evenly on both sides. Coat the top of the fillets with cooking spray.

Heat a large cast-iron skillet coated with cooking spray over medium-high heat. Add the fillets and cook, turning once, for 6 minutes, or until the fish flakes easily.

Makes 4 servings

Per serving: 204 calories, 31 g protein, 6 g carbohydrates, 6 g total fat, 1 g saturated fat, 54 mg cholesterol, 1 g fiber, 295 mg sodium

Health note: People with depression who take monoamine oxidase inhibitors (MAO inhibitors) should avoid alcohol and other fermented or aged products, such as the cheese in this recipe.

Cod Steaks Sicilian-Style
The Healing Factor: Excellent source of vitamin C and omega-3 fatty acids

1 tablespoon extra-virgin olive oil
1 medium onion, halved and thinly sliced
1 cup thinly sliced fennel
2 cloves garlic, minced
$\frac{1}{2}$ teaspoon dried thyme, crushed
$\frac{1}{4}$ teaspoon salt
$\frac{1}{4}$ teaspoon freshly ground black pepper
1 tablespoon balsamic vinegar (see note)
1 can (16 ounces) crushed tomatoes
$\frac{1}{2}$ cup orange juice
4 cod steaks (1$\frac{1}{4}$ pounds)

Preheat the oven to 425°F.

Heat the oil in a large nonstick skillet over medium-high heat. Add the onion, fennel, garlic, thyme, salt, and pepper and cook, stirring frequently, for 4 minutes, or until the vegetables are tender-crisp. Add the vinegar and cook for 30 seconds.

Stir in the tomatoes and orange juice and bring to a boil. Reduce the heat to medium-low and simmer for 5 minutes, or until the sauce is slightly thickened.

Place the cod steaks in a 9- by 9-inch baking dish. Spoon the sauce over the fish. Bake for 12 minutes, or until the fish flakes easily.

Makes 4 servings

Per serving: 221 calories, 28 g protein, 15 g carbohydrates, 6 g total fat, 1 g saturated fat, 61 mg cholesterol, 3 g fiber, 592 mg sodium

Health note: People with depression who take monoamine oxidase inhibitors (MAO inhibitors) should not use the vinegar in this recipe. Substitute orange juice for vinegar.

DESSERTS

Most people don't think of desserts as healing foods. Though the following recipes may not be as nutrient-dense as others in this chapter, they do supply their share of vitamin C and fiber. Besides, by ending your meals with these treats, you'll be less inclined to indulge in unhealthy sweets that supply lots of empty calories but nothing in the way of nutrition. So dig in—your taste buds will thank you!

Summer Fruit Compote

The Healing Factor: Excellent source of vitamin C and fiber

1 cup water

1 package (6 ounces) mixed whole dried fruit

3 tablespoons frozen orange juice concentrate

2 tablespoons packed brown sugar

3 whole allspice berries

1 bay leaf

1 stick cinnamon or a pinch of ground cinnamon

3 medium peaches, cut into ¾-inch wedges

3 medium plums, cut into ¾-inch wedges

1 cup pitted sweet white or red cherries (optional)

In a large saucepan, combine the water, dried fruit, orange juice concentrate, brown sugar, allspice berries, bay leaf, and cinnamon stick or ground cinnamon. Bring to a boil over high heat. Reduce the heat to low, cover, and simmer, stirring occasionally, for 10 minutes, or until the fruit is very tender.

Add the peaches and plums. Cover and simmer for 5 minutes, or until the peaches and plums are tender but not mushy. Stir in the cherries, if using, and cook for 3 minutes. Remove from the heat and place in a serving bowl. Let stand for at least 1 hour, or until the fruit has cooled and the flavors have blended. Remove and discard the bay leaf and cinnamon stick before serving.

Makes 6 servings

Per serving: 217 calories, 3 g protein, 56 g carbohydrates, 1 g total fat, 0 g saturated fat, 0 mg cholesterol, 7 g fiber, 5 mg sodium

Cooking tip: Once you've added the fresh fruit, don't let the mixture boil. Let the heat of the liquid gently cook the fruit. Boiling will make it break up.

Broiled Peaches and Strawberries

The Healing Factor: Excellent source of vitamin C and a good source of fiber

5 medium peaches, cut into 1-inch wedges

1 ½ pints strawberries, hulled and quartered

2 tablespoons honey

½ teaspoon ground cinnamon

⅛ teaspoon ground allspice or cloves

1 tablespoon butter, cut into small pieces

3 tablespoons slivered fresh mint, lemon verbena, or cinnamon basil (optional)

Preheat the broiler. Coat a large baking sheet with sides with cooking spray.

In a large bowl, combine the peaches, strawberries, honey, cinnamon, and allspice or cloves and toss to coat well. Place the fruit on the prepared baking sheet. Dot with the butter.

Broil, turning the pan 2 or 3 times (no need to turn the fruit), for 4 minutes, or until the fruit is glazed, bubbly, and golden brown in spots. Remove from the oven and let cool slightly.

Sprinkle with the mint, lemon verbena, or cinnamon basil, if using. Serve warm or at room temperature.

Makes 6 servings

Per serving: 111 calories, 1 g protein, 23 g carbohydrates, 3 g total fat, 1 g saturated fat, 5 mg cholesterol, 4 g fiber, 23 mg sodium

Pear and Almond Crisp

The Healing Factor: Excellent source of vitamin C

4 large pears, cored and sliced ½-inch thick

2 tablespoons maple syrup

1 tablespoon lemon juice

1 teaspoon vanilla extract

½ teaspoon freshly grated nutmeg

1 cup rolled oats (not quick-cooking)

⅓ cup sliced natural almonds

¼ cup packed brown sugar

2 tablespoons whole grain pastry flour

2 tablespoons cold butter, cut into small pieces

2 tablespoons canola oil

Preheat the oven to 350°F.

Combine the pears, maple syrup, lemon juice, vanilla extract, and nutmeg in an 11- by 7-inch baking dish.

In a medium bowl, combine the oats, almonds, brown

sugar, flour, butter, and oil and mix with your fingers to form crumbs. Sprinkle the topping over the pear mixture.

Bake for 40 minutes, or until the pears are tender and bubbly and the topping is lightly browned.

Makes 8 servings
Per serving: 271 calories, 4 g protein, 45 g carbohydrates, 10 g total fat, 3 g saturated fat, 8 mg cholesterol, 5 g fiber, 134 mg sodium

Strawberry Tart with Oat-Cinnamon Crust
The Healing Factor: Excellent source of vitamin C and fiber

Crust
⅔ cup rolled oats
½ cup whole grain pastry flour
1 tablespoon sugar
1 teaspoon ground cinnamon
¼ teaspoon baking soda
2 tablespoons canola oil
2 to 3 tablespoons fat-free plain yogurt

Filling
¼ cup strawberry all-fruit spread
½ teaspoon vanilla extract
1½ pints strawberries, hulled

To make the crust: Preheat the oven to 375°F. Coat a baking sheet with cooking spray.

In a medium bowl, combine the oats, flour, sugar, cinnamon, and baking soda. Stir in the oil and 2 tablespoons of the yogurt to make a soft, slightly sticky dough. If the dough is too stiff, add the remaining 1 tablespoon yogurt.

Place the dough on the prepared baking sheet and pat

evenly into a 10-inch circle. If the dough sticks to your hands, coat them lightly with cooking spray.

Place a 9-inch cake pan on the dough and trace around it with a sharp knife. Remove the cake pan. With your fingers, push up and pinch the dough around the outside of the circle to make a rim 1/4-inch high.

Bake for 15 minutes, or until firm and golden. Remove from the oven and set aside to cool.

To make the filling: Meanwhile, in a small microwaveable bowl, combine the all-fruit spread and vanilla extract. Microwave on high for 10 to 15 seconds, or until melted.

Brush a generous tablespoon evenly over the cooled crust. Arrange the strawberries evenly over the crust. Brush the remaining spread evenly over the strawberries, making sure to get some of the spread between the strawberries to secure them.

Refrigerate for at least 30 minutes, or until the spread has jelled.

Makes 6 servings

Per serving: 187 calories, 4 g protein, 31 g carbohydrates, 6 g total fat, 0 g saturated fat, 0 mg cholesterol, 3 g fiber, 65 mg sodium

Cooking tip: For a calcium boost, you can serve the tart with a scoop of fat-free vanilla frozen yogurt on the side.

PART V

They're Beating Arthritis—And You Can, Too!

Golf Keeps Her Up to Par

Hall of Famer Nancy Lopez plays too well to have what golfers call a handicap. But in 1999, she nearly acquired a handicap of a more serious sort: severe osteoarthritis of the knee.

"My doctor asked me how long I wanted to keep competing," recalls Lopez, who first swung a club at about the time most little girls are still swaddling their dollies. "A chill crept up my spine. I was playing in pain, but I was only 42."

Instead of surgery, she opted for a treatment called viscosupplementation. This treatment mimics synovial fluid, the lubricating liquid in healthy joints. Lopez's doctor injected the fluid into her knee three times to "grease" and cushion the joint. She was pain-free almost immediately—but not totally out of the rough.

"Osteoarthritis is a progressive disease," she notes. "It could get worse if I allow the muscles that support my knees to weaken." She's determined to keep those muscles strong and flexible with what she describes as a "baby and build" routine.

Every morning, Lopez stretches her quadriceps, the thigh muscles that stabilize the knees and thus reduce any pressure on the joints. Standing erect, she bends her right knee, gently pulls her heel to her butt, and holds for count of three. Then she repeats with her left leg.

To strengthen her quads, which can significantly decrease the risk and progression of osteoarthritis, Lopez performs sitting squats. Standing against a wall with a rubber ball between her knees, she bends her knees and slides her back down the wall until her thighs are parallel to the floor. She squeezes the ball, relaxes, then repeats 5 to 15 times.

Note: If you have osteoarthritis of the knee, check with your doctor before doing these exercises yourself. You want to be sure your knees are up to the challenge.

Sopranos Star Orders a "Hit" on Her RA

Emmy-nominated Aida Turturro plays Janice Soprano in HBO's critically acclaimed series *The Sopranos*. Off-screen, however, she's one of the more than 2 million Americans who suffer from rheumatoid arthritis, a chronic disease characterized by inflammation of the joints. In that role, she's more accustomed to enduring pain than to doling it out, Cosa Nostra–style.

"As a kid, I just sort of hung in there," says Turturro of the persistent pain in her hands, feet, and knees that can range from crampy to excruciating, depending on the day. "But as I got older, I became more aggravated with the disease, more impatient. And only then did I think I might be able to minimize my symptoms, not simply put up with them."

Today Turturro does both. She walks 20 to 30 minutes a day to keep her joints limber and her muscles strong. She stretches religiously, practices yoga regularly, eats healthfully, and experiments with drug-free pain relievers such as acupuncture. "It took a long time," she says. "But I finally realized, nobody's gonna take care of me but me."

A Physician Heals Himself

Halsted R. Holman, M.D., has spent the past 40 years researching and treating rheumatic diseases—and the past 10 years suffering from osteoarthritis himself. Both experiences have convinced him that the key to successfully dealing with chronic joint pain just may be in the hands of the patients themselves. It's called self-management, and it works.

"Any technique that you can use on your own to better control your disease is considered self-management," explains Dr. Holman, professor of medicine at Stanford University. "Engaging in exercise and relaxation to reduce pain, adopting practical strategies for navigating daily activities, addressing the social consequences of chronic pain—all of these qualify as self-management." For his part, Dr. Holman plays tennis on weekends and faithfully uses the stationary bike and strength-training machines at his gym during the week to control his joint pain.

As medical adviser for the Arthritis Foundation,

Dr. Holman felt motivated to help develop a course on self-management after 10 years of research revealed that people who were proactive about relieving their joint pain experienced significant improvement. "We didn't make them better physiologically," he explains. "But something as simple as helping them overcome their fear of exercise led to more physical activity, less pain, and less need for doctor visits."

The 18-week course conceived by Dr. Holman and his colleagues, with support from the Arthritis Foundation, is called Connect & Control. Participants learn the latest methods for relieving pain, strategies for reducing stress and depression, and the most effective uses of medication, nutrition, and exercise. They also get daily updates, e-mail reminders, and personalized diet and exercise advice and support.

For more information on Connect & Control, call your local Arthritis Foundation chapter or visit the organization's Web site at www.arthritis.org.

Fighting Arthritis One Crunch at a Time

Doyt Conn, M.D., starts each day with 100 sit-ups. This wouldn't be so remarkable if he were a U.S. Marine. But he's not a gunnery sergeant. He's a doctor, and he has osteoarthritis of the spine.

"There's a myth that arthritis is something you can't do anything about," says Dr. Conn, senior vice president of medical affairs for the Arthritis Foundation. "I do sit-ups every morning to maintain my muscles—especially my abdominal and large back muscles."

Dr. Conn is passionate in his belief that people with any type of arthritis are not powerless against their pain. "There's no question that you can help yourself with exercise," he says.

"If you become sedentary, you'll rapidly lose muscle mass and mobility," he explains. "The arthritis process may accelerate." On the other hand, if you can handle an easy-does-it fitness routine, you can minimize your pain and increase your range of motion. That way, you'll stay a step ahead of your arthritis symptoms.

She Gives Arthritis a Peace of Her Mind

Like her mother, Lois Hazel has osteoarthritis of the spine. But unlike her mother, this 57-year-old publishing professional from Kintnersville, Pennsylvania, is using yoga as a gentle antidote to her symptoms. The benefits have been even greater than she anticipated.

When Lois was in her late forties, her back pain drove her to an orthopedic surgeon. He advised physical activity to strengthen the muscles that support her back and to increase her flexibility. At the time, Lois was looking for an outlet from her stressful marketing job. She also was trying to reign in her high blood pressure. Yoga seemed like a good way to achieve all those things.

After trying a beginner's Sivananda yoga class at a nearby fitness center, Lois immediately fell in love with it. Like all yoga disciplines, Sivananda emphasizes breathing, relaxation, and correct posture. The stress relief came almost immediately. "After the first class, I could have slept like a baby, yet I felt renewed and calm," she says. "It was the most amazing thing I had ever experienced—like a super drug with no bad side effects. I went back again and again. And I've never been disappointed."

Every once in a while, Lois has a flare-up, which is common with osteoarthritis. "It feels like a giant hand reaching in and squeezing my spine very, very hard," she says. "The pain can literally take my breath away." For relief, she stops whatever she's doing and takes a few minutes to practice yoga breathing and check her posture. The improvement is always noticeable.

Yoga also helped lower her blood pressure. "And it was a godsend when I had oral surgery," she says. "I calmed myself with yoga breathing, and that helped me get through the procedure with minimum stress."

To manage her arthritis, Lois complements her yoga therapy with daily walks and an occasional over-the-counter pain reliever. She also does abdominal exercises to strengthen the muscles in her lower back, which support her spine.

According to Lois, taking up yoga was one of the best health decisions she ever made. "When the pain hits, if I just remember to breathe and concentrate the breath into my spine, it absolutely works," she says. "I can feel that giant hand softening, relaxing its grip."

Lois is determined to avoid the pain her mother lived with. "She was severely debilitated by arthritis in her later years, and I don't want to end up the same way," she says. "Yoga is helping me take a different path."

Learning a Lesson from Broadway Joe's Knees

Quarterbacks take a beating on the field, and Joe Namath certainly was no exception. Today the former New York Jets star suffers from osteoarthritis of the knees, spine, and thumb as a result of years of twisting, turning, stopping, and starting on the football fields he called home for most of his young life.

"Football is a great sport, but the body wasn't designed for it," says Namath, who retired in 1977. He had both knees replaced in 1992, which allowed him to lift his two young daughters without fear of falling down. The surgery also took away the pain, which was "always there, always in the back of my mind," he says.

Today Namath lifts weights and works out on an elliptical exercise machine, a combination stairclimber and cross-country skiing device that goes easy on his knees and spine.

Arthritis will get worse if you don't take care of

your body, he warns. "I know that changing habits is hard, especially for people who haven't worried about diet or exercise for most of their lives," he says. "But it's not impossible. You have to make it a priority."

He Took the Plunge—And Avoided Surgery

After he was diagnosed with arthritis in 1996, Roger Sizoo did exactly what his doctor ordered. Sort of. He took his pain medicine. But those stretches and flexibility exercises his doctor wanted him to do? Well, they got lost in the daily shuffle.

Within 6 months, Sizoo, a retired executive from southern California, couldn't bend over to pick up his morning paper. He had trouble even putting on his socks and tying his shoes.

"I was in real pain because I didn't have any flexibility in my joints at all," Sizoo recalls. "I was in pretty tough shape." In fact, it got so bad that he told his doctor to go ahead and schedule hip-replacement surgery.

But then, with his daughter's encouragement, Sizoo enrolled in an aquatic fitness program at a local YMCA. The 60-minute water workouts three days a week, combined with flexibility exercises every day, did wonders. Soon Sizoo's surgery was scrubbed, and the only painkiller he needed was an occasional aspirin.

"Life has taken on a new dimension," Sizoo says. "I sleep better. I feel better. I'm more flexible and mobile than I've been in years, and I don't feel any pain.

"You can take control of your arthritis. You don't want to roll over and feel sorry for yourself. You want to do something about it if you can."

She's a True Survivor

She runs, swims, and rides a Harley. And through 6 weeks of competition on the hit CBS show *Survivor*, she ate a worm, braved the Australian outback, and out-strategized 15 other wannabes to become the million-dollar winner.

But what's most remarkable about Tina Wesson, a mother of two and nursing assistant from Knoxville, Tennessee, is that she does it all with rheumatoid arthritis (RA).

Tina had been diagnosed with RA, a serious disorder involving inflammation of the joints, 8 years before her *Survivor* stint. "It hit me—bang!" she recalls. "I had been playing tennis, and when I got out of my car, everything hurt."

Her pain was so bad that she slept sitting up and couldn't get out of the bathtub by herself. She had swelling in her hands, wrists, and knees. Just shrugging hurt her shoulders.

Prescription arthritis drugs controlled her condition

so well that she had only two painful flare-ups in 7 years. Since returning from the remote *Survivor* camp—where she ate little more than rice (plus the occasional worm) and competed by (among other things) swimming the crocodile-infested Herbert River—Tina has had what she describes as "a little bit of trouble." But while she was there, she says, "I felt awesome as far as the RA was concerned. My friends in the outback didn't even know I had it."

With her Earth Mother disposition and *Steel Magnolias* drawl, Tina was popular with her teammates and with many—though not all—of the show's fans, who posted a weekly play-by-play on the Internet. But she admits to being stung by accusations on some sites that anyone who can win racquetball tournaments, run a marathon, and survive *Survivor* must be lying about having RA.

"There's a misconception about RA," she explains. "There are varying degrees of arthritis. Some may hear RA and think minor joint discomfort; others think crippling deformity. I do realize that mine is not a really severe case." Yet Tina has not been pain-free since that moment when she could barely get out of her car. "It's at a point where I can tolerate and live with it," she says. "But if I had my legs cut off, I would be calling the Paralympic Games tomorrow. I am that type of person. I will push past pain."

Tina strives to educate people about arthritis. She has this advice for others who share her disease: "See a doctor right away; don't suffer through it! Find something that works for you and lets you lead a semi-normal life. Be active to the point of your ability," says the woman whose goal is to "live the life less ordinary."

An Olympian Fight Against Pain

Anyone who has ever played the game Twister knows that a split isn't pain-free. Yet gymnast Bart Conner, who was diagnosed with osteoarthritis more than two decades ago, can still do one—and with arguably less pain than when he was in his prime.

"As an athlete, you think that pain is a normal, inescapable part of your life," shares Conner, who grabbed a pair of Olympic gold medals in 1984. "It was only after I retired that I woke up to my condition (osteoarthritis in his left elbow, right knee, and lower back) and realized the absolute need to stay ahead of my pain through medication, exercise, and intensive stretching.

"When you're hurting, you don't feel like moving," explains Conner, who is married to fellow former Olympic gymnast Nadia Comaneci. "Yet activity is exactly what people with arthritis need the most. If you don't exercise, your muscles grow even weaker.

So you have more grinding, bone on bone, and increased pain."

In addition, many sedentary people put on weight, which places more pressure on their joints and produces more pain. As a result, they're even less inclined to work out.

The trick, according to Conner, is to stay ahead of the pain curve so you can keep moving. "Pain isn't noble," he says. "It isn't even normal. It's debilitating, and I urge you to work very hard with your doctor to get rid of it, not endure it."

PART VI

Resources

For More Information

Thanks to the Internet, learning about arthritis has never been faster or easier. But you need to be sure you're getting your information from sources you can trust. The following list can steer you in the right direction. All of these organizations are reputable and on the cutting edge of arthritis research.

American College of Rheumatology
Web site: www.rheumatology.org
Telephone: (404) 633–3777
Offers educational materials and publications, including journals and a monthly newsletter, that cover all aspects of arthritis. The Web site features a search tool for finding a rheumatologist in your area.

American Juvenile Arthritis Organization (AJAO)

Web site: www.arthritis.org
Telephone: (800) 283–7800

A council of the Arthritis Foundation (see below), AJAO addresses the special needs of children, teens, and young adults with rheumatic diseases. Offers a variety of helpful products and services.

Arthritis Foundation

Web site: www.arthritis.org
Telephone: (800) 283–7800

Publishes *Arthritis Today* magazine, and offers books, videos, and free brochures through its online store. The Web site also features a search tool for locating chapters and events in your area.

Centers for Disease Control and Prevention (CDC)

Web site: www.cdc.gov
Telephone: (800) 311–3435

Maintains a wealth of statistical and epidemiological information on an array of diseases, including arthritis.

National Institute of Arthritis and Musculoskeletal and Skin Diseases (NIAMS)

Web site: www.niams.nih.gov
Telephone: (301) 495–4484
(877) 22–NIAMS (226–4267)

A branch of the National Institutes of Health, NIAMS supports arthritis research as well as training for scientists who conduct the research. Visit the Web site to print fact sheets and order information packets.

Index

**Eat Peanut Butter Every Day and Lose
All the Weight You Want!**

The Peanut Butter Diet

Holly McCord, M.A., R.D.
Nutrition Editor, *Prevention* Magazine

Recipe Coordinator, Regina Ragone, M.S., R.D.,
Food Editor, *Prevention* Magazine

You *can* eat peanut butter every day and still lose weight!
Many health-conscious dieters have shied away from this
tempting treat, but new studies show that peanut butter
can actually lower your risk for heart disease and diabetes
and help you shed unwanted pounds. And because THE
PEANUT BUTTER DIET is so satisfying, those who follow it are more successful at slimming down than those
who choose a traditional low-fat diet:

Dig in and discover:

- *50 fast-and-fabulous recipes*
- *4 weeks of delicious, super-easy meal
  plans*
- *A day-by-day diet you can stick to—even
  when you're eating out*
- *Fitness strategies to boost your
  metabolism and decrease body fat*
- *Special tips and treats for the whole
  family*

**AVAILABLE WHEREVER BOOKS ARE SOLD FROM
ST. MARTIN'S PAPERBACKS**